Infant Feeding and Nutrition for Primary Care

Donald Bentley MB, DCH, MSc, FRCP, FRCPCH
Consultant Paediatrician
Former Honorary Clinical Senior Lecturer
Imperial College of Science, Technology and Medicine, London

Sophie Aubrey BSc(Hons), DipD, SRD
Chief Paediatric Dietrician
Barts and The London NHS Trust, London

Melissa Bentley MBBS, BSc(Hons), MRCS
Specialist Registrar
The Royal National Throat, Nose and Ear Hospital, London

Radcliffe Medical Press
Oxford • San Francisco

Radcliffe Publishing Ltd
18 Marcham Road
Abingdon
Oxon OX14 1AA
United Kingdom

www.radcliffe-oxford.com
Electronic catalogue and worldwide online ordering.

British Library Cataloguing in Publication Data

A catalogue record for this book is available from the British Library.

ISBN 1 85775 866 8

Typeset by Aarontype Ltd, Easton, Bristol
Printed and bound by TJ International Ltd, Padstow, Cornwall

Contents

Foreword

I am privileged to be the mother of four children and grandmother of seven and to have worked in general practice/primary care for over 40 years. Hence, I thought that I knew everything that was required concerning infant feeding and nutrition. However, I was mistaken, as this book has taught me a lot and will, I am sure, be invaluable to GPs, health visitors and also, indirectly, to patients.

Obviously in a review of a book of more than 140 pages a brief foreword cannot cover all the topics included. Hence, I have selected a few areas of particular interest to me, but this should not imply that other areas are of lesser importance. I am convinced that the interests and needs of the many who will purchase this book will be varied but fully rewarded by reading it.

In Chapter 1, 'Breastfeeding and human milk', it was disappointing to find how much Great Britain lagged behind New Zealand, i.e. 69% versus 84%, but reassuring to read of the protective effect of breastfeeding against diabetes. Many will be surprised that all can breastfeed, including grandmothers and young girls. I was less convinced of the link to a possible reduction in the risk of cot deaths but encouraged that even if the mother inadvertently lies on top of her baby while breastfeeding in her sleep, the baby is able to move its head and avoid asphyxiation. We know that some food allergies are transmitted in the breast milk, but the risk of eating peanuts when breastfeeding is again rightly emphasised.

It was useful to read about breast pumps and to have the contact details of their makers. Other important contacts include The National Childbirth Trust, the La Leche League and the British Association of Perinatal Medicine.

Each paragraph included useful lists.

I personally felt that Chapter 5, which deals with vegetarian diets, was especially relevant to my family as we have two vegetarian daughter-in-laws who have produced between them three healthy breastfed babies. The same chapter also includes the major religious cultures and the dietary restrictions associated with them. However, some of these diets may present potential problems for infants, especially during the weaning period.

Formula feeding is dealt with in great detail. There are excellent appendices dealing with energy intake, fluid requirements, protein intake and growth charts for infants at different ages and stages.

The increasing importance of the feeding of premature and low birthweight babies is dealt with in detail, including the various strategies used in their weaning. There is a comprehensive list of vitamins and a full discussion emphasising the danger both of deficiencies and of excess vitamin consumption.

The book also deals with possible gastro-intestinal problems, including abdominal migraine and non-enteric problems. The relationship of feeding problems to disease conditions in later life are emphasised and especially the avoidance of obesity and dental decay.

The book finally deals with topical nutritional issues, including genetically modified foods, BSE and the risks of immigrant communities. Every chapter has excellent references for further reading and additional useful tables giving extra information.

It is a book that no practice should be without and, hopefully, this will be the case in the majority of progressive practices.

Lotte Newman CBE, FRCGP, FRNZCGP
General Practitioner
Past President of the Royal College of General Practitioners
February 2004

Preface

We believe that there is a need for a book that endeavours to answer the many nutritional-based questions that parents may want to put to their family doctor or health visitor. Parents may well know instinctively how to nurture their infants, but controversies over nutrition require information for informed decision-making. Our joint clinical and nutritional experience has shown that time and again the same controversial topics cause unnecessary concern, if not anxiety. There is a glut of information with which we are all bombarded by the media. Yet much of the dogma we both hear and read is made without any scientific foundation and is often highly contentious. Examples of such confusing issues include the role and safety of soy milks where there is a family history of allergy. Is there a place for goat's milk? Are vitamins really essential? As infant weaning foods are invariably salt-free, sugar-free and additive-free, what does a mother do when preparing her own food for a toddler which will contain salt, sugar, etc., and does it matter?

There is an increasing recognition of the relationship between early feeding patterns and subsequent health problems in later childhood and adulthood. We know now of associations between fetal and infant nutritional status with subsequent cardiovascular disease as well as diabetes. It is cogent to note the words of the new National Service Framework for Children: 'Healthy children have more chance of becoming healthy adults'.

No book on this topic can claim to be totally objective and solely based on science: the fact is that we know too little to be didactic in many areas. However, this represents the considered opinions of people with a great deal of experience in this field.

In this our latest book, a consultant paediatrician with a particular interest in nutrition and gastroenterology has combined forces with a paediatric dietitian and a trainee consultant, to look at the many aspects of nutritional care that confronts parents from day one of parenthood. We have endeavoured to encompass important aspects of breastfeeding, with inevitable mention of HIV/AIDS; choice of baby formula; allergy (eczema, asthma, etc.) and its prevention; hyperactivity; obesity; prevention of heart disease; unconventional (exotic) diets; role of probiotics; and many other major topics – which at times bewilder the expert, let alone the mother.

More elaborate details can be found in our first book on paediatric nutrition, *Clinical Nutrition in Paediatric Disorders* (Bentley D and Lawson M. Balliere Tindall, 1988), and, more recently, *Pediatric Gastroenterology and Clinical Nutrition* (Bentley D, Lifschitz C and Lawson M. Remedica Publishing, 2002), but in this new text we have focused on the many dilemmas posed by the very basic yet controversial subject of feeding a baby or infant and allied topics.

Acknowledgements

We wish to acknowledge the support and advice of Drs NJ Meadows, N Hasson, C Michie, J Nathan, M Pampelli, Gina Boakes and Andrew Ward of Remedica Publishing. We are particularly indebted to Alyson Colley, who is both our former and present editor, and to our mentor Arlene Seaton. The cartoon drawings are by Rosemary MacManus – former ward sister to Donald Bentley.

We owe a debt of gratitude to Dr Carlos Lifschitz, Associate Professor, Baylor College of Medicine, Houston, our former co-author, and Dr Margaret Lawson, Nestlé Senior Research Fellow, Childhood Nutrition Research Centre, Institute of Child Health, London, who was the co-author of our two earlier textbooks.

CHAPTER 1

Breastfeeding and human milk

In most – yet not all – circumstances, the best possible food for an infant is breast milk. Health workers have a responsibility to encourage a mother to breastfeed her baby, and to support her with information and skilful assistance, given she is not vehemently antagonistic to such a positive proposal. A global and constant effort must be made to protect, promote and support breastfeeding, which can be a matter of life and death for babies.

About 15–20 years ago, breastfeeding rates in New Zealand and Great Britain were similar. Since then, however, although the rate in New Zealand has risen to approximately 84%, the overall level of mothers breastfeeding at birth in the UK has stayed at about 69% (Infant Feeding Survey, 2000). Furthermore, this equates to those infants put to the breast at least once – by four months, only 28% are still being breastfed; by eight months, a mere 16%. In Sweden, an information and education programme resulted in a doubling of the number of mothers lactating within a period of only five years: from 31% in 1972 to 62% in 1976–77. A similar programme in New Zealand of specialist lactation nurse consultants (known as Plunket nurses), akin to health visitors in the UK, now see over 90% of infants under one year of age. Although the reasons for such improvement in New Zealand are multifactorial, the key role of specialist lactation nurse consultants and Plunket family centres must have formed a major component of this successful breastfeeding programme in one part of the Antipodes.

The late Professor DB Jelliffe, an international authority on human milk, pointed out that in some communities, if a mother died in childbirth, her newborn was buried with her because of the hopelessness of a baby deprived of its mother's milk. According to the World Health Organization (WHO), every year over a million babies die for want of breastfeeding. Even where clean water and sanitation are available, artificially fed babies are at greater risk of disease and death. Breast milk will facilitate the opportunity for an infant to realise his or her full potential for health and growth.

Yet babies are remarkably adaptable creatures who can grow adequately on many mixtures of foods, and have always done so. We have all met happy babies who have been artificially fed, just as we have all encountered hungry babies being badly breastfed who benefited from being given additional food. But we cannot deny that all these babies are at greater risk than is the happily thriving breastfed baby. We would be disingenuous with parents if we said that their choice was not risky and had no potential for later adverse effects on their child's life. However, despite advice from the expert, many parents weigh up the risks of artificial feeding and choose to go ahead with it regardless, driven by a number of motives. Other mothers will begin breastfeeding and experience difficulties that make them consider weaning; for lack of appropriate support and help, many will wean too early.

Why breastfeed?

Many books and papers elaborate on the complex and fascinating role of human milk in infant health and development, and perhaps even adult health and disease, too. There are many compelling factors that influence the informed parent to choose breastfeeding.

Benefits for the baby

For the baby, breastfeeding:

- provides nutritional and growth benefits
- optimises neurological and intellectual development
- enhances the immune system and increases resistance to certain infections
- reduces the incidence of gastroenteritis (e.g. rotavirus, polioviruses, etc.)
- reduces the risk for some chronic diseases (e.g. infectious and allergic disorders of alimentary and respiratory tracts)
- reduces the incidence of necrotising enterocolitis in preterm babies (presence of epidermal growth factor)
- may reduce the risk of 'cot death' (sudden infant death syndrome) and 'near-miss cot death' (acute life-threatening events)
- reduces the risk of obesity
- contributes to proper mouth and jaw development – breastfed infants tend to have a reduced incidence of cavities and need fewer orthodontic corrections later in life
- optimises hand-to-eye coordination
- provides emotional benefits – most breastfed babies cry less because they are held more.

Antimicrobial and antiviral factors in breast milk

There is some evidence in human newborns of a phenomenon known as 'closure', in which the lining of the small bowel becomes mature and does not absorb proteins or toxins. There is even some evidence to suggest that, occasionally, this bowel-wall maturation can develop within the intestine before birth. Until this radical change arises, the infant is at risk of allergen sensitisation (*see* Chapter 8).

There is in breast milk a unique and special antibody known as 'secretory immunoglobulin A' (SIgA). SIgA, which is derived from immunoglobulin A, coats the bowel lining to inhibit microbes from sticking to the gut wall and also prevents the absorption of substances (e.g. antigens) that have a major role in the development of allergy. Professor Allan Walker, a distinguished paediatric gastroenterologist at Harvard Medical School in Boston, has aptly likened this property to that of an antiseptic paint which coats the bowel wall, and this analogy does portray the extraordinary characteristics of SIgA (Fig. 1.1).

Apart from the crucial antibodies to be found in human milk and the passive transfer, *in utero*, of other antibodies from mother to foetus, the immune systems do not develop competently for at least three to four months in the newborn. This

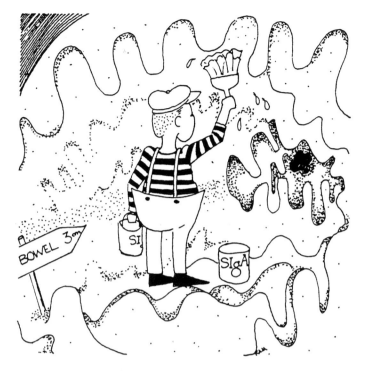

Figure 1.1   Secretory immunoglobulin A.

is why the recommendation to mothers is to breastfeed for at least four months and not to wean before then, so avoiding the exposure of a vulnerable bowel to potentially harmful foods.

If, for any reason, 'foreign' proteins, toxins or other harmful agents imbibed by a baby are 'allowed' to cross the bowel-wall lining, they will enter the circulation and may cause mild or severe symptoms. Alternatively, the portal of entry might be the nose, upper or lower airways, skin or eyes, and cause a local or a general-ised reaction. The 'foreign' agent or antigen is not identified as 'self' and so elicits an inflammatory reaction. It does not matter if the foreign body is a transplanted kidney or an invading virus: the principal features of the response will be the same. This initial inflammatory reaction will be succeeded by a variety of immune activities because of the existence of several classes of antibody and cellular properties.

The body endeavours to contain the reaction and engulfs the invading agent prior to elimination. To do this, specific types of blood cells and other highly specialised cells in certain parts of the body (for example, the bowel wall itself) become actively involved in the response triggered by the arrival of a 'foreign' or invading protein or protein-like particle. A combined effort by the antibody and sophisticated body cells destroys or inactivates the antigen and so recovery takes place. If the baby is re-exposed to the same antigen at a later date, a further reac-tion occurs. However, if the antigen is not successfully dealt with, symptoms appear. These will depend upon the site – for example, in the outer layers of the eyes (conjunctivitis), in the skin (eczema), in the nose (hayfever), in the lungs (asthma), and in the bowel (diarrhoea, windiness, colic or gut bleeding).

There are a number of additional components in human milk that help fight infection. For example, human milk contains living cells such as neutrophils, which will themselves destroy bacteria, whilst others (lymphocytes) have the ability to form antibodies. In addition, human milk contains the enzyme lysozyme and the iron-binding protein lactoferrin. Lysozyme damages the wall of certain bacteria, thereby destroying these microbes (Fig. 1.2). The lysozyme content of human milk is 3000 times that of cow's milk. Lactoferrin competes with particular bowel micro-organisms (bacteria and yeasts) for free iron, which is needed for their growth (Fig. 1.3).

Furthermore, the milk contains enzymes that not only break down fat but can also kill a specific and common parasite – *Giardia lamblia*. This protozoa causes diarrhoea by temporarily damaging the cells that line the absorptive surface of the bowel wall. Consumption (via ingestion of contaminated food or water) of as few as ten cysts can produce illness in both children and adults. If untreated, it results in severe weight loss and other problems. Giardiasis is often found in overcrowded communities with poor sanitation. However, it is not an infrequent cause of diarrhoea in the UK, and, indeed, many other developed countries. Epidemics in day nurseries have been reported.

Diarrhoea is globally uncommon in those who breastfeed. However, even in developed countries, annual and recurrent bouts of diarrhoea are seen frequently. In the UK, from autumn to spring, there are many hospital admissions because of gastroenteritis – frequently due to viruses such as the rotavirus, small round structured virus (SRSV) or adenovirus. We must not underestimate the disruption to family life when one of the members has an acute hospital admission. Furthermore, following discharge, the baby or infant's behaviour will take time to settle down. The consequences to the child of such experiences should encourage us to advocate prolonged breastfeeding. In the UK, and indeed in many other countries, the rotavirus is a major cause of diarrhoea, yet breast milk is rich in antibodies to this viral agent. A thriving child will not be at severe risk from viral enteritis; however, in the developing world, a combination of sudden diarrhoea and malnutrition will often cause death. This topic is inevitably of greater importance in the

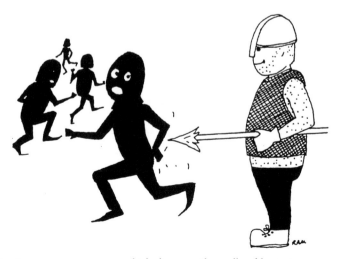

Figure 1.2   Lysozyme: an enzyme which damages the walls of bacteria.

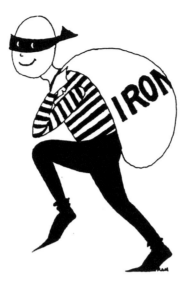

Figure 1.3   Lactoferrin.

poorer nations, where the astronomical death rate and consequences of diarrhoea can be associated with the use of formula.

It is not just bowel disease that is less common with human-milk feeding: many prevalent chest infections due to specific viruses would be seen less frequently had the mother breastfed. The American Sedgwick documented as long ago as 1921 the protective effect of breastfeeding against chest infection as well as diarrhoea.

As can be seen, the protective agents in human milk are very numerous. Furthermore, it has been shown that if a mother is exposed to any infection, in some circumstances her own milk will develop specific antibodies to that infectious agent. While each year scientists struggle to identify the flu virus and make a vaccine before the next winter, every breastfeeding mother exposed to the flu virus has made protective antibodies within days of exposure and is feeding them to her baby.

Protection against diabetes

Recent evidence has shown that, where there is a family history of diabetes, the potential risk to a baby within such a family can be very considerably reduced by breastfeeding. Researchers have demonstrated that prolonged breastfeeding – and, most importantly, the total avoidance of any milk formula until seven months – will reduce the likelihood of future diabetes by as much as 50%. Even offering 100% human milk for just three months, again excluding all baby milk, is beneficial in terms of decreasing the probability of future diabetes. This awareness will put greater pressure upon all healthcare workers in these circumstances to discourage mothers from offering baby formula.

Benefits for the mother

For the mother, breastfeeding:

- increases calorie expenditure, making it easier to lose the pounds gained during pregnancy

- contracts the uterus (due to release of repeated bursts of oxytocin), which reduces the flow of blood after delivery and protects the mother from post-partum haemorrhage
- delays the return of normal ovulation and menstrual cycles
- reduces maternal mortality
- preserves haemoglobin stores
- reduces the risk of premenopausal breast cancer and, possibly, ovarian and uterine cancers
- promotes bonding between mother and child
- helps relaxation
- saves time and money.

Prolactin is a hormone that is formed in the pituitary gland in response to suckling (and emotional factors), then travels, via the bloodstream, to the breast, where it stimulates and sustains milk production. Prolactin also serves to inhibit the response of the ovaries to follicle-stimulating hormone (FSH), which is responsible for ovulation. Consequently, the return of ovulation is delayed in lactating mothers, thereby reducing the likelihood of a further pregnancy. However, despite the folklore tales on this topic, breastfeeding cannot be regarded as a reliable technique of suppressing fertility.

The degree of protection derived from breastfeeding relates to several factors – frequency of feeds and length of time on the breasts, as well as the question of complementing with cow's milk formula. All influence the competence of breastfeeding as a contraceptive. Lower levels of prolactin are noted, for example, when the mother provides only a limited number of breastfeeds as opposed to practising unrestricted breastfeeding. These relative reductions in circulating levels of prolactin permit ovulation to occur because the ovaries are not inhibited in their response to FSH.

Furthermore, during lactation, levels of prolactin decrease despite continued breastfeeding, and, by the tenth week, the mother will ovulate. Mothers need to be reminded that 5% will ovulate before they menstruate and, paradoxically, some will have menstrual cycles during which they fail to ovulate. Early supplements with formula and reduced suckling will result in lower levels of prolactin and a greater likelihood of ovulation, with a risk of conceiving. Theoretically, a mother solely breastfeeding in an unrestricted style might not require any method of contraception in the initial 10 weeks. However, because of the many variables – such as the baby feeling unwell and then not being an active suckler for a period of time – this advice must be tempered with considerable caution.

The close visual and physical contact that is part of the breastfeeding pact can only cement the relationship ('bond') between mother and her baby (Fig. 1.4). Fortunately, however, this 'bonding' is not exclusive to those fed on breast milk, and we have met countless contented babies given only formula but well united with their mothers.

Societal benefits

For society, breastfeeding:

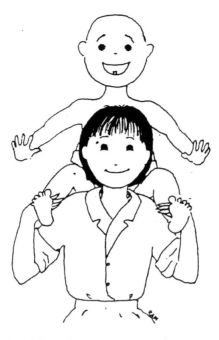

Figure 1.4 Mother–baby relationship.

- reduces total medical care costs for the nation – breastfed infants typically need fewer sick care visits, prescriptions and hospitalisations
- reduces pollution of air, water and land from production of artificial baby milk and its packaging
- conserves energy sources.

Who can breastfeed?

Many mothers are surprised to learn that virtually any woman can breastfeed a baby, given the infant is put to the breast often enough to stimulate the flow. A woman who adopts a baby and wants to breastfeed can do so even though – and this is regrettable – she has not been able to adopt in the early days of life but perhaps has had to wait weeks before she is presented with her baby. Grandmothers, schoolgirls and childless women have all been able to make a success of lactation if they are both well motivated and patient. Small breasts are no less able to store and express milk than are larger ones. Initially, the empty breast will frustrate the baby, so expert support and self-confidence play a role in achieving a good outcome. At times, a woman might decide after the baby is some weeks old that she wants to give up the use of fomula and try her own milk. Allergic reactions might have become evident and some wise health visitor or midwife has astutely related the symptoms to the milk formula; thus, the mother has revised her earlier opposition to breastfeeding. We have even observed mothers who initially having decided their baby was to be adopted, subsequently changed their minds and, with much courage, breastfed. This has arisen even when early physical separation occurred and the mother was conditioning herself to giving up her baby.

When not to breastfeed

Sadly, there are a number of circumstances in which lactation must be avoided. These include mothers in developed countries with HIV infection. Furthermore, if a mother is suffering from an active psychotic disorder and is fearful of harming her newborn, or has 'open' active tuberculosis in her lungs, then clearly formula is a safer option. The presence of anti-cancer agents such as cyclophospamide, cyclosporine, doxorubicin or methotrexate in the breast milk constitutes a contraindication, as does maternal lithium, cocaine, heroin or marijuana use. Refer to the extensive list in the Breastfeeding Appendix of the British National Formulary (BNF) No. 44.

Why do so few mothers breastfeed?

It is sobering and most disappointing to note that, in the UK, the Office of Population Censuses and Surveys (2000) reported a rise in breastfeeding of only 2% since 1980, with 69% of all newborns being breastfed a minimum of once after birth, and only 21% still being breastfed at six months. Moreover, there are dramatic social class differences, which have always given much cause for concern – 85% of mothers with higher occupations breastfeed, compared with only 52% of those with no occupation. The mother's level of education is also closely linked to her likelihood of breastfeeding. For example, 64% of mothers in the highest educational category were breastfeeding at six weeks, compared with 27% of mothers in the lowest educational group. It is tempting to link the higher rate of infection in the disadvantaged classes with suboptimal breastfeeding patterns.

An obvious area where professionals should make more intensive efforts to persuade mothers to review their plans for a formula-feeding practice is in the antenatal period, and not when the baby has appeared and the mother has had many months in which to develop an entrenched and antagonistic attitude to lactation. Reports have shown that in the UK, only half of first-time mothers were questioned antenatally about their feeding intentions. Also, too little is done in schools, and how many countries have educational television advertisements at prime time, demonstrating the benefits of human milk? Mothers opposed to lactation are strongly influenced by their own mothers, who perhaps have had a distaste for breastfeeding, demonstrating a biased attitude which is easily propagated. Fathers in the lowest occupational categories (e.g. manual workers) generally do not favour the idea of their wives or partners breastfeeding, but frequently have not met the experts to discover the plus points of lactation. Perhaps evening antenatal clinics and joint appearances (mother plus father, or, for the single isolated parent, mother plus a friend or grandparent) would help remedy this depressing picture.

Composition of human milk

Breast milk is the most complete form of nutrition for the majority of infants (Fig. 1.5). A mother's milk in normal circumstances has the right type and amount of fat, carbohydrate, water, protein, vitamins and minerals that are needed for a baby's growth and development. Most babies find it easier to digest breast milk than they do formula.

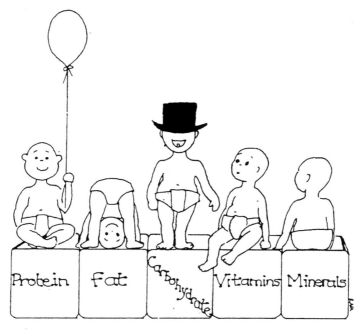

Figure 1.5   The composition of human milk.

The composition of human milk is an interesting – and, indeed, surprising – topic, in that there is variability in content between colostrum, transitional milk, and mature foremilk and hindmilk, differences between each breast, and also alterations on a daily basis.

Colostrum

Colostrum is the initial milk produced in the early days after birth and, because of its protective properties against infections, has a vital role to play in maintaining good health.

Often we hear mothers – and, indeed, inexperienced professionals – underemphasise the enormous importance and benefit of early breast milk. Sadly, it is frequently regarded, quite inappropriately, as water, because it is thin and translucent. However, it is rich in immunoglobulins, including IgA, which has a key role in the prevention of disease, and antibody formation against viruses and bacteria. Before the end of the first week, it will be replaced by transitional milk, which has a different composition. It is salient to record that colostrum, although containing less fat than mature milk, is rich in protein, electrolytes and vitamins. Moreover, this highly specialised milk contains a particular enzyme that prevents the breakdown in the gut, by digestion, of protective antibodies.

It is a matter of interest and perhaps relevance to note that in some hoofed animals and other species, colostrum plays such a major role in disease prevention that its absence is associated with fatal infections. At times, farmers give it to particular calves to protect them.

Mature milk

The transition to mature milk is gradual and stimulated by frequent suckling. The composition of mature breast milk is not homogenous, but varies between individuals, each breast and during a feed.

Protein
The protein in breast milk comprises:

- casein (curd)
- whey (non-casein) proteins – including lactalbumin, lactoglobulin, IgA etc.

Human milk has a lower casein content than cow's milk. When casein meets the acid within the stomach, it will form curds. Infant-milk manufacturers now produce whey-dominant milks, to avoid the formation of such casein curds.

Importantly, minute quantities of ingested proteins from the cow have been identified in human milk. These potential allergens are derived from the maternal diet and may have a role in sensitising the baby and the development of adverse food reactions.

Fat
Fat is made up of triglycerides, which can be broken down into fatty acids. Some fatty acids are 'saturated' and others 'non-saturated'. Although breast milk contains both saturated and unsaturated fats, the latter are present in higher concentrations. The fatty acid content of human milk is related to the maternal diet.

Fat content varies during a feed, being low at the start ('foremilk') and increasing as the feed progresses ('hindmilk'). As a result, the fat concentration in hindmilk is double that in foremilk. Furthermore, there is a change in fat composition of a feed during the course of a day.

Within human milk, but not cow's milk, there is the enzyme lipase, which breaks down the fat so that it can be absorbed from the bowel.

Human milk is rich in the essential fatty acids linoleic acid and alpha-linolenic acid. These can be converted into long-chain polyunsaturated fatty acids (LCPs) – arachidonic acid and docosahexanoic acid, respectively – which are required for brain and retinal development.

Carbohydrate
The sugar in both human and cow's milk (as well as in all other non-specialised formula milks) is lactose. During digestion, it is broken down into glucose and galactose. Galactose has a major role as a constituent of myelin (part of the sheath that surrounds nerve fibres).

Vitamins and minerals
All of the important vitamins, both fat-soluble and water-soluble, are present in human milk, e.g. vitamins A, D, E, K, C and B. Although levels of vitamins D and K are thought by some experts to be inadequate, well-nourished babies born at term are unlikely to become vitamin-depleted if the mother has an adequate vitamin/ mineral status. However, we believe it is prudent to give vitamin supplements to the mother if her diet is marginal, and all breastfed infants should have vitamin drops from six months of age.

The let-down reflex

Milk is secreted continuously into the alveoli of the breasts, but milk does not flow easily from the alveoli into the ductile system and therefore does not continually leak from the breast nipples. Instead, the milk must be 'ejected' or 'let down' from the alveoli to the ducts before the baby can obtain it. This process is caused by a combined neurogenic and hormonal reflex called the let-down reflex (or draught reflex/milk ejection reflex) involving the hormones oxytocin and prolactin (Fig. 1.6).

When the baby suckles the breast, sensory impulses are transmitted to the pituitary gland, resulting in the secretion of oxytocin and prolactin. The oxytocin

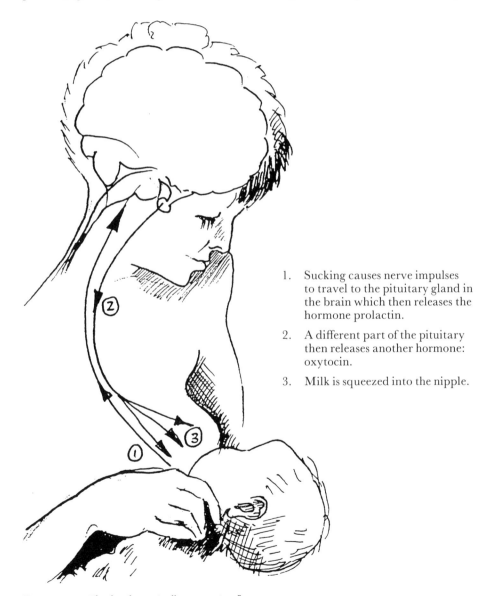

1. Sucking causes nerve impulses to travel to the pituitary gland in the brain which then releases the hormone prolactin.

2. A different part of the pituitary then releases another hormone: oxytocin.

3. Milk is squeezed into the nipple.

Figure 1.6   The let-down (milk-ejection) reflex.

then flows in the blood to the breasts, where it causes the tiny muscle cells (myoepithelial cells) that surround the milk glands to contract, thereby expressing the milk from the alveoli into the ducts which are behind the nipple. Thus, within 30 to 60 seconds after a baby begins to suckle the breast, milk begins to flow.

Suckling on one breast causes milk flow not only in that breast but also in the opposite breast, hence the drip milk from the other side.

Successful breastfeeding is not dependent solely upon stimulation of the nipples; sight, sound and also thoughts about the baby will act as stimuli for the let-down reflex.

Timing of the first feed

Because of the let-down reflex mechanisms, early breastfeeding (i.e. immediately or one to two hours after delivery) has been shown to correlate well with successful lactation in the following weeks. Sight and close contact with the baby facilitates hormone release, thus enabling the mother to discharge milk from the nipples when suckled. Stress can impede this ejection reflex (*see* p. 11); therefore, we should endorse a policy of not separating mother and newborn in the delivery suite, nor in the immediate postnatal period. Another disincentive for the estab- lishment of breastfeeding is a caesarean section under general anaesthesia rather than a spinal block. A local anaesthetic would at least ensure that the mother was fully alert and so could put her baby promptly to the breast if she so wished. How- ever, highly motivated mothers or equally determined midwives can diminish the counterproductive influence of an anaesthetic on successful lactation.

Caesarean section is a major operative procedure. The subsequent pain from the mother's abdominal wall is such that the intention to carry out lactation needs to be a resolute one. Should the mother need painkillers in the postoperative period, this might impede her efforts to successfully breastfeed. Because of the scar and discomfort, the position when suckling is critical – unless the baby is being sup- ported and held away from the site of the incision, it will not be easy to relax. If the baby is fed whilst the mother is in bed on her side, she will need physical assistance when she switches to the other breast. After the first week, pain and discomfort from the wound will be lessened and successful feeding is more likely to become established. A kindly midwife can all too readily block a mother's endeavours to lactate by endorsing too generous a use of analgesics and sedatives, but, above all, by the misplaced yet well-meaning practice of not awakening mother at night. In maternity units with a high caesarean section rate, more intensive efforts to achieve a successful policy of lactation will be needed than in other centres where such sections are less frequent.

In some maternity units, a standard dose of pethidine, or a comparable drug, is given for the relief of pain, which is not related to the mother's stature, i.e. if the mother is six foot tall and weighing 90 kg, she will inevitably need more medi- cation than a thin, diminutive 'ballerina' type. Also, often to avoid the vomiting that can accompany the use of opiates (e.g. codeine, morphine, pethidine), older- type anthistamines are given. These can sedate the mother and impede her effort to breastfeed, because of her reduced state of alertness and responsiveness to the baby's presence. After the delivery, the antenatal drugs might still be active and keep mother in a sleepy and unaware condition, perhaps for many hours.

Rooming-in of mother and baby is most important if we are to see any likelihood of breastfeeding becoming established. Happily, nowadays, few maternity units have the end-of-ward nursery seen until recently in too many hospitals. Every evening the cribs were wheeled away from the mother's bedside and not returned until the following morning. No doubt many mothers cried silently and their babies more vociferously.

Mother and baby separation can be the result of the newborn having to enter an intensive care unit (ICU), perhaps for ventilation or other specialised therapy. However, even in this situation – and allowing for the fact that the newborn may be hidden beneath extensive monitoring equipment within an enclosed, or perhaps an open, crib – we believe it is not necessary to separate the baby. One of us (DB) was staggered recently to hear a ward sister on a neonatal ICU with an international reputation, telling her medical colleagues that the mother of a ventilated newborn would not need to be with her baby. We are strongly critical of such advice. However, we realise that few nurses or paediatricians need reminding of the enormous importance of keeping mother and baby together in all situations whenever possible, unless mother poses some hazard to the baby, such as being mentally very ill, perhaps psychotic or physically threatening to her baby – but this is not common.

With goodwill and a positive professional attitude, mother and baby can, and should, be kept close together physically and not just visually. After all, even if apparatus and tubes are blanketing the baby, there is invariably some part of the baby's bare skin, be it just the forehead or foot, that gives the mother the opportunity of touching the skin and hopefully making eye contact. Kangaroo care is where mothers nurse their infants against their chests, being held within the mother's shirt or top, to facilitate skin to skin contact even when the baby may be quite ill. This technique has become increasingly popular in some special care units.

Unfortunately, there are situations where mother and baby cannot always be together. For example, one of us (SA) had twins prematurely: one was in special care while the other was being ventilated in intensive care – therefore it was physically impossible to be with both newborns.

When mothers are unable to breastfeed, they should be encouraged to express very frequently – at least three-hourly and a minimum of once during the night. If the milk supply appears to be diminishing, the mother should be advised to express more often. A photograph of the baby or an article of his or her worn clothing close to hand may help stimulate milk production. It is also important that the mother eats and drinks plenty.

Technique of breastfeeding
Breastfeeding position

Comfort and position are important in the establishment of successful breastfeeding. The baby should be supported snugly in the crook of the mother's elbow. Sitting up, especially in a traditional narrow hospital bed, can often be a most difficult way in which to nurse a baby. A better alternative might be for the mother to lie flat in bed on her side with the baby; and the less clothing between mother and baby, the easier it is to feed.

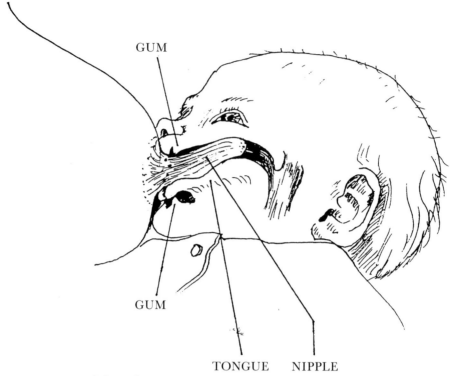

Figure 1.7 How a baby sucks.

For breastfeeding to be successful, the whole nipple (including the areola area at the nipple base) must be placed well within the mouth (Fig. 1.7). Understandably, a mother who is relaxed physically and mentally will have her milk flowing with less impedance than one who is tense and stressed. Also a multigravid woman will be less troubled than a primigravida. If the baby's mouth is pushed onto the nipple, the activation of the important rooting reflex will result in the baby turning towards the cheek that was touched and so stimulated by a primitive mechanism. Frequently a baby will root towards the bedclothes or nightwear that incidentally touched one cheek, thereby disrupting an established feeding session. When the nipple is well within the mouth, it should be directed upwards as if being aimed at the baby's nose. Once the let-down reflex is active, the baby ought not to come off the breast.

It is important to recall that milk reserves are stored beneath the areola and so need to be emptied. In situations where the areola is very large, yet must be emptied, it can be compressed by finger and thumb to ensure it is flattened. Finally, we need to remind mothers both to empty their breasts completely, and to alternate the side they offer.

Breastfeeding during sleep

There is much mythology and superstition about the entire topic of breastfeeding, but certainly particular anxieties exist in respect of a mother feeding in bed and suffocating the baby by overlying during sleep. Mothers have been observed – and, indeed, filmed – whilst sleeping, and it is quite possible for baby to suck at the breast whilst mother sleeps peacefully throughout the entire exercise. If the mother inadvertently positions herself on top of the baby, her newborn will move his or her head around and so not become asphyxiated from the breasts, whatever their size. Parents can also be reassured that, in normal circumstances, the baby will not fall out of bed. However, as a result of a recent European study into cot deaths, the Foundation for the Study of Infant Deaths has changed its guidelines. Bed or couch sharing could be unsafe for infants in the first eight weeks of life.

Our only other reservations relate to when a mother is ill, is on medication such as tranquillisers, antidepressants or antipsychotic agents, or is under the influence of alcohol. An alert and physically well mother who is uninfluenced by drugs or psychological illness will encounter no problems, and, when awakened, will have satisfied both the baby's nutritional needs and her own sleep requirement. For some basic reflex mechanisms to work, the infant's cheek needs to make contact with the bare breast, and then, in response, the baby's mouth will open and 'home in' on the nipple. Observe a frustrated, if not crying, baby, fully clothed, endeavouring to find the nipple, perhaps through the mother's bra or other obtrusive underwear blocking access. A naked mother and unclothed baby, given neither are cold, readily dovetail, and feeding at the breast is facilitated.

Length of time at the breast

The cornerstone of advice can be condensed into the simple message of 'little and often' and there should be no place for clocks. Between three and four minutes at a breast will release 80% to 95% of the milk, depending upon many factors, such as the absence of anxiety, fatigue or emotional/physical stress during lactation. Within the first two minutes, 50% of the milk can be released. To reassure the mother that timing at the breast is irrelevant, ask for her views about lactation in the developing world. There, for example, a mother may feed her baby whilst working in the fields, and, not surprisingly, is unconcerned about 'x' minutes at each breast. Fortunately, she is unlikely to have a watch or clock. The kidneys of the newborn, especially the immature baby (i.e. less than 37 weeks at birth) have not evolved to cope with large intakes of protein infrequently – thus, small volumes and often is what is needed.

The ideal volume of milk

One of the many major benefits of milk from the breast is that we do not know what volume the mother is giving her newborn – and this is just how the situation should be. A well mother who wants to successfully feed her offspring from her breasts will, if given advice and support, invariably succeed.

Frequency

Newborns may need to be fed one to two-hourly, having as many as 8–10 feeds a day. At one month, feeds will be every two to three hours, and by two to three months of age, every four hours.

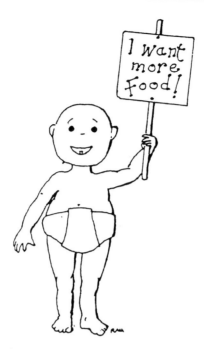

Figure 1.8 'Demand' feeding.

The act of suckling stimulates the nipple and surrounding area; consequently, messages are sent to the pituitary gland to cause the release of the hormones prolactin and oxytocin. Prolactin controls milk production within the breasts, and so we can see quite readily that the more the baby suckles, the greater is the volume of milk formed. Presumably, the more frequent the feeding, the higher is the efficiency of the let-down reflex (*see* p. 11).

The more intensive the activity of 'demand' feeding, the better the actual supply of milk (Fig. 1.8). To achieve an improved weight gain, when the midwives and doctors are concerned about a baby not thriving, the simple remedy is to put the baby to the breast more often. Tight schedules of feeding must be abandoned and the baby fed often, and that could indeed mean every one or two hours. It can be appreciated that for unrestricted but successful feeding, telling the mother to put the baby to the breast four-hourly will thwart baby and mother, and ensure failure of the mother's endeavours. The commonest reason given by mothers for cessation of breastfeeding is that they believed they had insufficient milk. This sadly is a false belief and is demoralising for mothers. The simple remedy is for them to feed more frequently and not to resort to complementary feeding, which is counterproductive.

Often, mothers are given conflicting advice about their lactation practice; this can be very confusing, particularly for a vulnerable mother with her first baby.

Case study

Davina's mother was told that her baby's poor weight gain was due to insufficient breast milk. However, she was feeding four- to six-hourly in a baby only seven days old who had not returned to her birth weight of 3 kg.

The family doctor rightly advised that the baby be breastfed every two to three hours and even at night. Davina's father helped by giving the baby expressed breast milk that had been stored in the fridge during the previous 24 hours. This ensured that Davina's mother had six to eight hours of sleep and so felt revitalised for daytime activities, when she could focus on her baby's needs. Within three days of the new management plan, Davina started to thrive and gained 8–10 g/kg/day.

Energy consumed and stools

During the first few months, most infants need 100–115 kcal/kg/day. This equates to 150–180 ml of breast milk per kilogram per day (based on actual weight). If the infant does not thrive, the volume of milk should be increased. As discussed previously, this can be done by increasing the frequency of feeds or offering both breasts at a feed.

Stool character and frequency

Mothers, especially those in the UK and the US, are often overly concerned with the colour of the baby's stool, and their observations give them much unnecessary anxiety.

The early stool after birth is black and sticky as a result of the presence of meconium (debris, etc. from the bowel wall), but when milk passes along the bowel lumen, stool colour and consistency will change. The nature of a feed (i.e. human milk, cow's milk, soy milk, etc.), and the presence or absence of jaundice and phototherapy, all influence the characteristics of the stool.

In the healthy breastfed newborn, the stools are soft, odourless, and although usually yellow, may be green. Coloration depends upon the type and quantity of bile pigment present in the stool and is unimportant in the absence of biliary tract or hepatic disease.

Babies fed solely on breast milk never pass hard stools and do not get constipated. Initially, some of these babies may pass stools after every feed, resulting in eight or so nappy changes per day; however, others will pass only one stool on alternate days. After a few weeks, the baby's motions appear less often. Because breast milk is absorbed so efficiently, it is not surprising that babies fed solely on human milk produce so few stools. If the baby is well and thriving, this observation is of no significance. Underfeeding may be associated with frequent and small motions.

In contrast to those who are on breast milk, babies fed on formula produce stools that are firmer and brown, with an unpleasant smell. Also, formula-fed babies commonly pass stools less frequently than do those being suckled.

Weight gain

All babies who are born at the appropriate time with a normal weight for their sex lose weight after birth and then regain. This should not be true for those who were not nourished adequately *in utero*: they should not lose at all but slowly gain weight. A baby who is tube fed may have a more precipitous gain than one on the breast, because the appetite is bypassed and not used to determine uptake. A breastfed baby might not return to his or her birth weight until as long as 10–14 days after birth. The precise gain is not important, but weekly trends do matter. One baby may gain 25 g a day; another, 30 g – providing the baby is well, the practitioner need not be concerned. After four months, the velocity of growth is less, so the daily gain will drop to about 20 g.

Junior doctors, midwives and health visitors can easily get the mother too tuned in to the precise weight as opposed to the rate of gain and overall trend. We often need to remind mothers that using scales at several centres (baby clinic, GP's consulting rooms, hospital clinic and ward) gives dissimilar readings. Clothing might well be different at the time of each attendance. Similarly, measuring a baby's length, and also head circumference, will vary with the skills and patience of different personnel: on occasion, our nurses have reported a length that tells us a baby has shrunk. Nevertheless, plotting all babies' weight, length and head circumference regularly on the Child Growth Foundation growth charts is the best way of monitoring nutritional adequacy. The Child Growth Foundation have also produced new 'breast from birth' charts – weight charts specifically designed for breastfed infants. These charts recognise the different growth pattern of breastfed infants. Breastfed babies initially gain weight more rapidly, but from two or three months of age their weight gain decreases and they begin to move downwards across the centiles unless they are plotted on these new 'breast from birth' growth charts. The Child Growth Foundation argue that the new charts will prevent mothers and health professionals from becoming anxious and changing the infant from breast to formula milk when growth begins to slow down. The Child Growth Foundation also suggest the charts could be used as the reference for all British babies whatever the means of feeding.

Mother's diet and medication use during lactation

Lactation, in contrast to pregnancy, imposes a greater energy and fluid requirement. The additional energy needs for lactation are derived as increments, depending on the volume of milk the mother is producing. This ranges from 450 additional kilocalories per day in month one to 570 kcal per day for exclusive feeding in months three to six. There is no evidence to suggest that a gradual maternal weight loss, in part from uterine involution during lactation, is detrimental to milk production, but it is not advisable to follow a weight-reducing diet until after weaning. In principle, a mother's diet ought to be both well balanced and adequate; where this is not so, milk is produced at the expense of maternal tissue. Women can form milk containing adequate protein, fat, carbohydrate and most micronutrients even when their own sources are limited. Only prolonged lactation in nutritionally depleted women is likely to have an impact on milk composition: in these circumstances, the content of calcium, folate, and vitamins B_6, B_{12}, A and D may be reduced. The maternal diet will, however, affect the fatty acid composition of the milk, particularly that of LCPs, which are important for brain and retinal development (*see* p. 10).

We need to be concerned about the mother's calcium requirements, which rise to a staggering 1350 mg per day whilst breastfeeding: this is not achieved by even two pints of milk alone. In lactating young women and adolescents who will not have achieved maximum bone density, it has been suggested that daily calcium intake should be 1500 mg (three pints of milk). Milk and milk products play a vital role in mothers achieving their calcium requirements; if, for any reason, they are unable to include such in their diets, they require at least 1000 mg of calcium per day as a dietary supplement

There are also increased requirements for protein, vitamin D, thiamine (vitamin B_1), riboflavin (vitamin B_2), nicotinic acid (vitamin B_3), folate, and vitamins B_{12} and A. Vitamin D requirements are doubled to 20 μg/day. There has been a recent resurgence of interest in this due to the apparent increase in the incidence of rickets, particularly in inner-city Asian communities. New recommendations have suggested that pregnant and lactating women be given a supplement of vitamin D (*see* Chapter 6). The other increased requirements can easily be met by a varied diet.

If a lactating mother takes in caffeine-containing drinks or foods, the baby might become irritable or restless. Caffeine is present in tea, coffee, chocolate, cocoa and cola drinks. Alcohol also readily passes into breast milk and high intakes should be avoided during lactation.

Maternal fluid intake does not affect the volume of breast milk produced, but a lactating woman needs to consume more fluid – about two litres per day – to protect herself from dehydration. In practice, breastfeeding mothers are extremely thirsty and often take additional fluids.

Rarely, maternal medications can have a harmful effect on the baby; however, this is uncommon, and only if a mother takes specific treatment for serious diseases, such as cancer, blood clotting disorders, arthritis or thyroid disease, might we then discourage breastfeeding. Box 1.1 gives examples of drugs that can be found in human milk. It is all too easy for an inexperienced midwife or junior doctor to tell a mother to abandon breastfeeding because of his or her own ignorance about the influence upon the baby of the mother's medication. In the final analysis, it is sometimes possible to measure medical drugs that appear in the mother's milk and thus allay everyone's anxiety. However, for technical as well as economic reasons, it is not always easy to measure the medication within human milk.

Box 1.1   Maternal drugs contraindicated in breastfeeding.[*]

Bromocriptine	Amphetamine
Cyclophosphamide	Cocaine
Cyclosporine	Heroin
Doxorubicin	Marijuana
Dextroamphetamine	Nicotine
Ergotamine	Phencyclidine (PCP)
Lithium	
Methotrexate	
Phenindione	

---

[*] This list is not comprehensive.

Environmental pollutants such as DDT and isotopes (e.g. iodine, strontium and caesium) can be detected in the soil, then the grass upon which cows graze, and finally within the cow's milk which is ingested by lactating mothers.

Adverse (? allergic) reactions to food products in mother's milk

It has been known for some years that dairy foods ingested by a mother can be detected in her own milk. In earlier generations, there was a belief that what a mother consumed could influence the baby's health and behaviour. These impressions, if not superstitions, were noted, but not until immunologists were able to demonstrate the presence of cow's-milk proteins in breast milk did clinicians pay heed to such comments.

Many substances, foods, chemicals, pollutants (e.g. pesticides) and, of course, a number of medications find their way into the lactating mother's breast. It was in 1918 that Talbot in America reported the development of eczema in a baby after a mother who was totally breastfeeding ate a lot of chocolate. Even before birth, it is believed that the foetus can be sensitised to an antigen ingested by the pregnant mother.

A family history of eczema, asthma, hayfever, food intolerance or migraine would make the family physician suspect an adverse food reaction in a baby who is in discomfort following a breastfeed. The drug caffeine (present in cocoa, chocolate, coffee, tea, etc.) can be recovered from a lactating mother's milk and, as a stimulant, can distress an infant. The Committee on Toxicology of Chemicals in Food (COT) report on peanut allergy advises against the intake of peanuts for breastfeeding women.

Colic

We, in common with others, have at times observed the development of so-called colic in a baby being breastfed. Colic is characterised by vigorous, periodic crying episodes and bending up of the lower limbs, indicative of abdominal pain; the baby is more restless and distressed upon completion of a feed than at the beginning, when the baby presumably was hungry. We have been impressed that if mothers of such babies remove all milk and dairy products from their own diet, there is a sudden improvement in a high proportion of cases. In this situation, the mother must take a calcium supplement to ensure her requirement of 1350 mg/day is met. It is virtually impossible to achieve this level of intake without milk products in the diet.

If there is fresh blood in the stools of a non-constipated baby, milk-sensitive (or food-sensitive) colitis might be the cause (see Chapter 7). Usually, there is increased bowel activity with much flatus and borborygmi. In such cases, a paediatrician's opinion needs to be sought. The family practitioner will be rightly concerned lest the mother attributes the baby's pain and distress to colic, when a more serious condition such as bowel obstruction (e.g. an inguinal hernia incarceration, volvulus, etc.) is present.

Spices, garlic, beef, chicken and eggs, as well as other foods and drinks, in the lactating mother's diet can provoke problems in a small number of suckled babies – these foods, however, should not be avoided unless there is good evidence to do so.

Does avoidance of cow's milk and other allergens reduce the likelihood of eczema or asthma developing in the newborn?

There is much controversy in the medical profession about this, but a number of distinguished paediatric dermatologists and immunologists have shown the benefit of milk-protein avoidance in the early weeks and months of life. However, others have disputed this hypothesis. It would seem prudent, in the presence of a positive family history of intolerance to foods and when the bowel has an inadequate immune system (before four to six months of age), that the well-motivated mother is cautious and strictly avoids at least dairy products (Fig. 1.9). We do not believe that where one child has a history of allergy, the mother (if she has decided against breastfeeding) should resort to a soy milk (*see* p. 37), because that, too, can cause adverse reactions. Nor should she implement a diet that is low in antigens, at the time of weaning, unless eczema is evident and she has sought expert dietetic advice. Paediatricians, together with dietitians, must be involved in such decision-making by the parents.

There is a view that with a family history of significant atopy, probiotic (*Lactobacillus rhamnosus*) capsules should be ingested daily by a mother two to four weeks before delivery of the baby and given to the mother once a day whilst she breastfeeds. There is some evidence to show that probiotics will significantly reduce the presence and severity of eczema in such newborns.

Cow's milk can be found in many foods and it is not always an obvious ingredient; use the checklist in Box 1.2 as a guide to help avoid foods containing milk, where this has been expertly advised. Terms for milk products used in food labelling are listed in Table 1.1. Some medicinal preparations also contain milk products.

All those following a milk-free diet should be referred to a state registered dietician (SRD) to ensure there has been complete elimination of milk proteins and also to evaluate the calcium intake. Older infants who are not taking a substitute formula always require calcium supplementation.

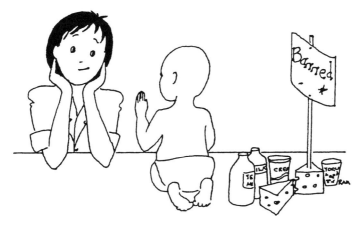

Figure 1.9 In the presence of a family history of allergy, some advocate the mother should avoid dairy products.

Box 1.2   Foods that may contain milk products.*

Protein foods	Sausages, burgers, frozen and canned meat and meat/fish in sauce, meat and fish coated in batter or breadcrumbs
Cereal products	Infant cereals, rusks, biscuits, cookies, bread, buns, cakes, pastries, canned spaghetti with cheese
Dairy products	Margarines; canned, dehydrated and frozen desserts and ice creams; canned and dehydrated baby desserts; powdered coffee whiteners and cream substitutes; malted milks
Fruits and vegetables	Canned and dehydrated vegetables in sauce
Confectionery	Milk chocolate; filled chocolates and chocolate bars; toffees and soft sweets or candies; lemon curd; chocolate-type spreads
Miscellaneous	Canned and dehydrated soups; mustard; pickles in sauces; flavoured crisps and similar snack items; salad dressings

---

* All ingredients should be checked for hidden sources of milk; many supermarkets now produce lists of milk-free products for their customers.

Table 1.1   Terms for milk products used in food labelling.

Buttermilk	Casein	Lactose	Milk solids	Whey
Butterfat, butter solids, milk fat, animal fat, artificial cream, artificial butter flavour	Caseinates, hydrolysed casein		Non-fat milk solids	Hydrolysed whey, vegetarian whey

Maternal problems associated with breastfeeding
Painful breasts (engorgement)

There are many potential problems that can arise during feeding of the newborn. When breastfeeding, especially if the breasts are not emptied frequently, tender and severely painful lumps can appear. To advise a mother then to stop putting her baby to the breast will only intensify the problem and is the wrong approach.

Our experience both within maternity units and in the community has convinced us that treatment of this very common problem can often be mismanaged.

Engorgement arises not only from the presence of excess milk but also may be the result both of an increased blood supply and leakage of lymphatic fluid from its vessels. Such leakage is secondary to the blocked blood vessels caused by the raised pressure within the breasts. The skin of the breasts appears shiny and has the features of orange-peel, with a pit-like surface. The lumps can be very conspicuous and discrete. This phenomenon is often linked with shivering attacks and the mother having a hot sensation; accordingly, doctors can readily interpret this situation as being due to a breast abscess, which is a different problem and requires medical treatment.

The main principles of treatment are to feed more often, and for longer periods of time. As Jelliffe reminds us: 'Successful lactation with an unimpaired let-down reflex leads to adequate emptying of the breasts without milk engorgement and less chance of nipple trauma.' Often it might be too difficult to suckle the baby because of swelling and tenseness, therefore some milk should be expressed (either manually or by a hand or electric pump) to soften the breasts. Applying icepacks will relieve both the tenderness and the pain, as will the use of hot or cold compression packs.

Nipple problems

Nipple soreness is one of the commonest reasons given by mothers who have abandoned lactation. It is disconcerting to recall that Mavis Gunther, a distinguished authority on the subject, said nipple soreness was almost entirely avoidable. She also wrote about 'psychosomatic' soreness. There can be no doubt that when a mother is anxious – or, indeed, ambivalent – about breastfeeding, and feels it is expected of her yet is reluctant to offer her own milk, nipple problems are commoner. We have often predicted on our ward rounds within the maternity unit which mother will have trouble with her nipples, even though they are perfectly normal in size and contour.

In common with so many topics in medicine, there are a number of theories as to why suckling a baby can cause sore nipples. If the nipple is not properly positioned within the baby's mouth, its lining can be damaged. Considerable negative pressure is created as the baby sucks, and if the nipple, because of its shape or length, is ill positioned, it will be injured and cause a painful stimulus for the mother. Examination of the nipple will reveal a line or bar composed of petechiae and small raised projections (papillae). With an adequate let-down reflex, the baby should not need to suck hard. When sore nipples are present, we need to review the mother's position and posture.

Sore nipples are said to be commoner in fair-skinned women with pinker nipples. A cardinal rule is that mothers should continue breastfeeding. Mothers often note that applying milk (especially hindmilk) to the nipple and allowing it to dry prevents soreness. We do not advise application of preparations on the nipple and areola, which is a sensitive site of skin, richly supplied with nerves. Lanolin, present in many skin preparations or creams that might be applied to lessen pain (e.g. analgesics or anaesthetic sprays), can cause skin reactions (e.g. contact dermatitis), and also reduce the 'pheromones'. These chemicals enable each baby to respond specifically to the unique odours of his or her own mother's nipples and so facilitate breastfeeding. Nipples need not be washed with soap and water. To be convinced of this advice, note the success rate of mothers breastfeeding in non-industrialised countries, who do not have such ready access to soap etc. and are not concerned with nipple preparation or hygiene.

If a crack appears, and this is not nearly as common as is thought, then it is important to try to express milk, because retention will lead to engorgement, and other problems can escalate, with eventual cessation of lactation.

In some women, nipples may be flat or even inverted. This may cause such women to feel disheartened as regards breastfeeding. However, it is uncommon for this apparent problem to pose as much difficulty as might be anticipated. The shape and protraction of nipples undergo a spontaneous and favourable change during pregnancy. Breast shells (shields), too, may help in this regard (Fig. 1.10). These devices consist of a plastic-saucer-like structure with a central hole in the inner surface. They can be worn antenatally inside a bra and exert pressure that may result in nipple protrusion, although there is no conclusive evidence that the shells do in fact achieve eversion of inverted nipples.

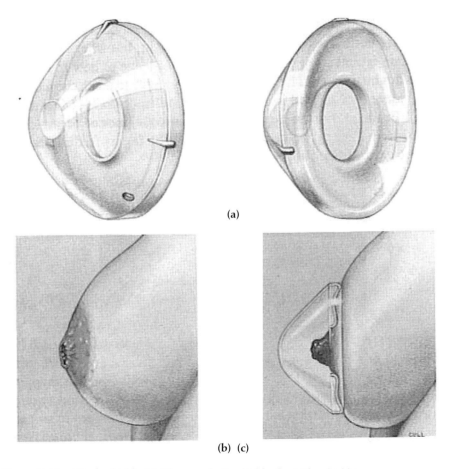

(a)

(b) (c)

Figure 1.10   Nipple shields. (a) Glass or plastic shields. (b, c) The shield in use.

Even if this apparent problem persists after delivery, it should not deter the woman from breastfeeding. We ought to remind such mothers that just as sexual excitability can transform flattish nipples into erectile structures, so can a suckling infant. Usually, pressure upon the areola will cause the nipple to extrude from its embedded position and so convince a mother that the baby will be able to latch on.

Jaundice and breast milk

Jaundice is a syndrome characterised by hyperbilirubinaemia and deposition of bile pigment in the skin, mucous membranes and sclera, with a resulting yellow appearance of the patient. Jaundice can be caused by a great many mechanisms.

A premature baby has a less efficient liver than one born at full term. The liver has a large number of tasks to perform. One important activity is for it to handle breakdown products of red blood cells. At the end of their lifespan (about 120 days), red blood cells rupture, releasing haemoglobin. The 'haem' element is reduced to form bilirubin, which binds to plasma proteins and is transported to the liver. Here, the bilirubin is removed from the protein and conjugated with glucuronate that makes it highly soluble, thus enabling it to be excreted in the bile. The immature liver in preterm infants is not efficient at conjugation.

Jaundice may appear in some breastfed babies, particularly those who are premature. Breast-milk jaundice is associated with raised amounts of non-esterified fatty acids (NEFA) in the milk. These fatty acids inhibit the transferase that conjugates bilirubin. Fortunately, this situation is not harmful and does not require treatment. Irrespective of the intensity of the skin's yellow colour, lactation ought to continue, even though such babies may be jaundiced for many days or even weeks.

Jaundice due to other conditions, such as ABO incompatibility or other causes of haemolysis, in contrast to breast-milk jaundice, might need light therapy (phototherapy). This may well prove very stressful to both mother and baby: the baby is separated from the mother, and then, naked and blindfolded, is put into an incubator and exposed to a light source. We believe that this technique is used too often and should not be authorised without an experienced paediatrician considering the clinical facts and then determining its validity in a particular case. If, phototherapy is deemed necessary, mothers should be prepared and emotionally supported. As with all situations, some mothers find the whole exercise less disturbing than do others. Because of the increased water loss from the heat created by the light bulbs, extra fluid is usually recommended, and the stool colour will alter and less-well-formed stools will be passed.

To convince a mother that her baby's jaundice is due to her breast milk, as opposed to unrecognised disease, some would suggest that the milk is withheld for 12–24 hours (expressed and saved), then later reintroduced. However, in our experience, this is counterproductive in that successful lactation can so readily be irretrievably disrupted. Measuring the infant's serum bilirubin serially and demonstrating it is mainly of an unconjugated (indirect) type will reassure the mother and her carers and help them to exclude the presence of obstructive biliary disease. The latter will be characterised by conjugated (direct) hyperbilirubinaemia and has serious connotations.

Expression and storage of milk

The baby's sucking reflex is not present until maturation reaches an age of 32–36 weeks (a normal 'term' delivery is 37–40 weeks). If this reflex is absent, sucking will not be activated when the nipple or teat of a bottle is positioned inside the baby's mouth. Therefore, until this age of development is achieved, a mother who wants to breastfeed will need to express her milk. This is then offered to the infant via a feeding tube passed through the nose and into the stomach.

Many contemporary women choose to express milk, via a hand or electric pump, to fit in with their lifestyles and work commitments. If a mother is working, particularly part-time, she could express her milk early in the morning or at any convenient time, and the carers of the baby use the expressed milk. Fathers or other carers often give a feed of expressed breast milk, particularly at night, so as to offer mothers a rest, get infants used to a bottle and for their own enjoyment. Expressing can also be a useful technique to increase milk supply – especially in the morning, when it is plentiful.

Furthermore, this option has a role in the most unlikely situation that the mother is on very powerful drugs (e.g. chemotherapy for cancer) which are present in her milk, the aim being that, when off treatment, she could return to, or indeed commence, breastfeeding. The milk pumped during therapy can be discarded. Other uncommon instances include a mother having 'open' and active tuberculosis, where, even after a short phase of anti-tuberculosis treatment, the infant can return quite safely to the breast, although he or she, too, will receive some of the anti-tuberculosis medication.

Before expressing milk, a mother needs to wash her hands carefully and practice acceptable techniques of hygiene. The milk container and pump must be kept clean and sterilised after use. Expressing milk by hand or pump can be a difficult and stressful exercise. A skilled midwife or counsellor is extremely important – and essential in the early phase.

Types of breast pumps

Hand pumps
The simplest and most compact of all hand pumps are the inexpensive types which can be bought from chemist shops or high-street baby-product sources. Because they are hand operated, they can be tiring, although a benefit is that the force of the vacuum and the speed of expressing is determined manually. However, for long-term use, the electric/battery pumps are often more successful.

Electric and battery-powered pumps
These are useful for long-term pumping where mothers frequently express. They require no manual effort and both the vacuum strength and cycle speed can be altered. Both single and double units are available. Suppliers include:

Egnell/Ameda Ltd
Unit 1
Belvedere Training Estate
Taunton TA1 1BH
Tel: 01823 336362
www.ameda.demon.co.uk

Medela
CMS House
Basford Lane
Leek
Stafforshire ST13 7DT
www.medela.com

It is often possible to hire such machines in the UK from some hospitals with maternity units, or from the La Leche League, or seek advice from the National Childbirth Trust (*see* p. 30).

Storage of milk

Breast milk can be kept at room temperature for six hours; in a domestic refrigerator for 24 hours or for three to five days if a temperature of 2–4°C can be guaranteed; in the freezer compartment of a fridge for one week; and in a deep freezer for three months. When collecting milk from the breast (or the 'drip' milk from the non-feeding side), we advise the use of plastic collecting bottles, if possible, because valuable and viable cells in the milk can be lost by sticking to the walls of glass containers.

Viruses in breast milk

Although, in general terms, bacterial parasites have difficulty surviving in breast milk, the RNA retroviruses, which include human immunodeficiency virus 1 (HIV-1) and human T-lymphotropic viruses 1 and 2 (HTLV-l, HTLV-2), use this route. Cytomegalovirus (CMV), Epstein-Barr virus and human herpesvirus 7 have been detected in human milk. This contrasts with hepatitis viruses B and C, which, although possibly being in relatively high viral numbers in the maternal circulation, are not frequently detected in milk.

Cytomegalovirus

CMV is a member of the herpes family. Breast milk is known to be a possible carrier of this virus. Depending upon the age and the immune status of the host, cytomegaloviruses can cause a variety of clinical syndromes (collectively known as cytomegalic inclusion disease), although the majority of infections are very mild and subclinical. The classic disease is congenital, being acquired *in utero* from the mother; infection can also be transmitted from mother to infant in passage through the birth canal or from ingestion of virus in the mother's milk. Fortunately, the majority of CMV infections in newborns are not apparent, and the baby is well. However, in some infected infants – albeit rare – there may be hepatosplenomegaly, jaundice, chorioretinitis, purpura, microcephaly, cerebral calcifications, and severe central nervous system sequelae with blindness, deafnesss, quadriplegia and mental retardation.

The situation is compounded by our ignorance, in that mothers are rarely screened to determine if they carry CMV. This is unsatisfactory, even though we do not have a vaccine. In the UK, the virus is present in 2%–6% of pregnant mothers and can be found in the urine of 1%–2% of newborns. In the US, it is thought that approximately 30 000 infants with CMV infection are born each year, and about one-tenth will have symptoms such as deafness and mild mental retardation. It has been shown in America that CMV infection is higher in women in the upper- and middle-income groups than in those with lower incomes. Furthermore, this infection is commoner at birth in the highly developed countries as compared with in the developing nations.

Hepatitis and breast milk

Some of the viruses responsible for hepatitis can be transmitted to the new-born from the mother prior to birth, at the time of delivery, or as a result of breastfeeding.

Hepatitis B
The hepatitis B virus (HBV) can be present in various body fluids of mothers. During the postnatal period, close contact between mother and newborn will facilitate transfer of the virus. Newborns of infected mothers from Asia or Africa are at particular risk of developing hepatitis B – more than three-quarters of the babies will develop the infection. The highest incidence is in children born to Chinese mothers.

Fortunately, transmission of HBV can be dealt with by the use of a special vaccine. Sophisticated markers of the disease exist (core antigen values) to measure the degree of risk of infectivity to those in proximity to the mother.

Hepatitis G
The hepatitis G virus (HGV), also known as GB virus C (GBV-C), an RNA agent, is transmitted mainly through the parenteral route. Approximately 2% of pregnant women are HGV antibody positive. There is a higher mother-to-infant trans-mission rate (30%–50%) of this virus than of HCV. A neonatal source can cause a persistent infection.

Breast milk and the HIV (AIDS) virus

More than 1600 children acquire HIV infection every day globally, and the majority as a result of mother-to-infant transmission. Fortunately, in the UK, policy changes and improvements in antenatal testing, perinatal antiretroviral therapy, planned vaginal or elective caesarean birth, as well as infant formula feeding, have dramatically reduced this transmission rate to less than 2% (Tudor-Williams & Lyall, 1999). In a study conducted in Uganda, a single oral dose of the antiretroviral drug, neviparine, given to HIV-infected women in labour, reduced perinatal HIV infection by about 50%. Additional data from this study demonstrated the continued bene-fit and safety of neviparine in reducing mother-to-child transmission of HIV up to 18 months, even in a breastfeeding population.

Between one-third to one-half of babies born to HIV-positive mothers are infected before or around the time of birth. A very significant number of cases worldwide have been caused by the virus being in the mother's milk, especially in the presence of mastitis or breast abscesses. It has been estimated that breast-feeding will confer an additional risk of 14% (95% confidence interval, 7%–22%) of mother-to-child HIV infection. Although some experts have disputed the evidence, it would clearly be prudent to note the warning issued by the Chief Medical Officer to the Department of Health and Social Security in the UK (April 1988 and July 1989). It is necessary to advise all mothers in the UK known to be infected with HIV to abstain from breastfeeding. Paediatricians in Africa have questioned the consequential hazards of such guidelines, since human milk is so protective against potential lethal pathogens. In most developing countries afflicted with AIDS, the hazards of bottle-feeding exceed the risk of mother-to-baby transmission of HIV infection. Women donating breast milk to pooled milk banks should be identified as being HIV antibody negative, although we must emphasise this does not give a 100% assurance that all is well. It is also important to note that if the pasteurisation technique is faulty, then HIV, if present, will not be destroyed.

Those at risk of HIV infection include:

* sexual partners of persons known to be infected with HIV
* men who have sex with other men
* anyone who has multiple sex partners
* anyone who has sex with a prostitute
* anyone who shares needles using illegal injected drugs
* anyone who exchanges sex for drugs or money
* anyone who has a sexually transmitted disease
* anyone who has had or currently has a sexual partner with any of the above risk factors.

> 'Behaviour changes can result in a decrease in new HIV infections in both rich and poor countries.'
>
> Arthur J Ammamann, President of Global Strategies for
> HIV Prevention, 2003

Support groups

There are those babies who seem trouble-free feeders, while others appear dis-heartened when fed, and readily cry, if not battle with the nipple and mother. At times, the explanation for this apparent conflict can be directed towards those responsible for the immediate postnatal midwifery management. A sudden surge of professional activity in a labour suite, which might well be modestly staffed, can result in insufficient time being offered to a mother keen to start breastfeeding. In such a scenario, we need to recall that the vital sucking reflex is strongest in the initial 20–30 minutes after birth, therefore the baby needs to be put to the breast within that unique first half-hour period.

Fortunately, many support groups exist, and with more openness on the part of midwives and maternity units, members of such groups, hopefully, are welcomed to counsel both mother and staff to ensure teaching is consistent, and the pro-fessionals do not contradict one another and confuse a well-motivated mother.

Sadly, but inevitably, many questions are put to our most junior doctors: some find it hard to admit that they know little of the art of lactation, and mothers sense the invalidity of the advice given. We would prefer to see each maternity unit or health centre have a single expert or a small group of 'nutrition' midwives who are committed, particularly in the antenatal period, to the propagation of breastfeeding.

Simple pieces of advice regarding position, type of chair, posture, skin-to-skin contact and creating a relaxed atmosphere, perhaps privacy for a shy mother, are all significant factors for the many who fail to establish successful lactation. Leaflets are available from voluntary organisations such as the National Childbirth Trust (NCT) and the La Leche League. Unfortunately, according to a UK study in 1985, as few as 5% of mothers use the expertise of such organisations.

National Childbirth Trust
Alexandra House
Oldham Terrace
London W3 6NH
Tel: 020 8992 8637
www.nct-online.org

La Leche League
BM 3424
London WC1N 3XX
Tel: 020 7242 1278
www.lalecheleague.org

La Leche League International
Post Office Box 1209
Franklin Park
IL 60131 - 8209
USA

The National Awareness Website
www.breastfeeding.nhs.uk

British Association of Perinatal Medicine
50 Hallam Street
London WIW 6DE
Tel: 020 7307 5640
www.bapm-london.org

Further reading

- Fry T (2003) The new 'breast from birth' growth charts. *J Fam Health Care.* **13**: 124–6.
- Hale T (2002) *Medication and Mother's Milk* (10e). Pharmasoft Medical Publishing, Amarillo, TX.
- Morgan J and Dickerson J (2003) *Nutrition in Early Life.* Wiley, Chichester.

CHAPTER 2

Formula feeding

The nutrition provided by modern formulas is adequate for a baby's growth and nourishment, and the choice from among the leading brands will ultimately be a personal one. The constituents of the various products are very similar and conform to the requirements of a Department of Health Special Committee on Infant Nutrition, and guidelines of the European Commission Directive, and the Codex Alimentarius body of the World Health Organization (WHO) and Food and Agriculture Organisation (FAO) (Table 2.1). There is no merit in the switching of formulas whenever a problem arises.

There is a strong recommendation from the Department of Health in the UK and the European Society of Paediatric Gastroenterology, Hepatology and Nutrition that, in the absence of a mother lactating, formula milk as the main milk drink should be continued until 12 months of age. Doorstep milk can be used in cooking only from four months of age. It is vital that formula or breast milk should provide the major source of milk until the infant is at least one year. Semi-skimmed milk can be used only in those over two years of age. Fully skimmed milk is unsuitable before the age of five years because of its low calorie and vitamin A content.

Standard infant milks

Most normal infant formulas are manufactured from heat-treated cow's milk that has been extensively modified, the aim being to bring the products as near as possible to the profile of human milk. Despite such extensive modification, however, it must be remembered that infant milk composition can only approximate that of breast milk. There are important, irreversible and fundamental differences, especially in the nature of the proteins, which were evolved for the calf: infant milks do not provide the immunological advantages of breast milk (*see* Chapter 1) and cannot mimic its changing composition during a feed and throughout lactation.

The commonest infant milks in the UK are still in powder form (for reconstitution with water) and sealed in a container with a scoop. More recently, ready-to-feed preparations have become available, in which the formula solution is in sealed cartons. These preparations, although more expensive than the powdered products, have the advantages of convenience and accuracy, as well as hygiene; as they inevitably involve less handling, the likelihood of introducing bacteria is reduced. Nevertheless, it is hoped that mothers will not be tempted to abandon breastfeeding in their favour.

Table 2.1 Recommendations for composition of infant formulas based on cow's milk – content (per 100 available kilocalories) for macronutrients and vitamins. From Bentley D, Lifschitz C and Lawson M (2002) *Pediatric Gastroenterology and Clinical Nutrition*. Remedica Publishing, London.

	EEC[1,2]
Energy per 100 ml milk	60–75 kcal (251–314 kJ)
Protein (g)	1.8–3.0
Taurine (μmol)	Minimum 4.2
L-carnitine (μmol)	Minimum 7.5
Nucleotides (mg)	Maximum 5
Lipid (g)	4.4–6.5
Linoleic acid (mg)	300–1200
α-Linoleic acid (mg)	Minimum 5
Linoleic/α-linoleic ratio	5–15
LCPUFA	
– n3	Maximum 1% total fat
– n6	Maximum 2% total fat
Carbohydrate (g)	7–14
Lactose (g)	Minimum 3.5
Sucrose (g)	Maximum 20% total carbohydrate
Vitamin A (μg retinol equivalents)	60–180
Vitamin D (μg)	1.0–2.5
Thiamine (μg) minimum	40
Riboflavin (μg) minimum	60
Nicotinamide (mg) minimum	0.8
Pantothenic acid (μg) minimum	300
Vitamin B_6 (μg) minimum	35
Vitamin B_{12} (μg) minimum	0.1
Biotin (μg) minimum	1.5
Folic acid (μg) minimum	4
Vitamin C (μg) minimum	8
Vitamin K (μg) minimum	4
Vitamin E (mg α-tocopherol) minimum	0.5

[1] EEC Commission Directive 91/321/EEC (OJ No L175, 4.7.91, p. 35).
[2] EEC Commission Directive 96/4/EC (OJ No L49, 28.2.96, p. 12).

To produce infant milks, cow's milk is modified as follows:

- reduction of total protein content, modification of the ratio of insoluble casein to soluble whey protein, adjustment of amino acid profile
- increase in carbohydrate (in the form of lactose and other sugars)
- adjustment of fat composition
- adjustment of vitamins, iron salts, minerals and trace elements.

Types of standard infant milks

Infant milks can be divided into two groups depending on ratio of casein and whey (two types of milk proteins) present:

- 'highly modified' (whey-based) milks, in which the casein:whey ratio is as in human milk, i.e. 40:60
- 'modified' (non-whey-based/casein-based) milks, in which the casein:whey ratio is 80:20.

Examples of each are provided in Table 2.2. Health professionals prefer the whey-based formulas as they are more similar to breast milk. There appears to be little advantage of one manufacturer over another. The formulas' labels and advertising material quite unjustifiably claim the casein-based formula is to satisfy the hungrier baby – to date, we have seen no published data that substantiate this assertion.

Nucleotides and long-chain polyunsaturated fatty acids

Nucleotides:

- aid the elongation of fatty acids into long-chain polyunsaturated acids
- promote T-lymphocyte development and increase natural killer cell activity
- promote the growth of so-called 'beneficial' bacteria, which play a role in competing with potentially pathogenic micro-organisms.

Because of their immunogenic properties, nucleotides are added to some infant formulas.

Long-chain polyunsaturated fatty acids (LCPs) – particularly docosahexanoic acid (DHA) and arachidonic acid (AA), both present in breast milk – are essential components of cell membranes within the central nervous system and retina. These fatty acids have been recommended recently, by a workshop of nutritional scientists, to be added to infant formulas for both term and preterm babies. Currently, most manufacturers have added LCPs to their term formulas; however, none of the therapeutic formulas except SMA High Energy have them included.

Table 2.2   Commercially available standard infant milks.

Manufacturer	'Highly modified' (whey-based) milk	'Modified' (non-whey-based/ casein-based) milk
Wyeth	SMA Gold	SMA White
Cow & Gate	Premium	Plus
Milupa	Aptamil	Aptamil Extra
Farleys	First Milk	Second Milk
Boots	Formula 1	Formula 2

Follow-on milks

These are special formulas that have been devised by the manufacturers to constitute part of a weaning regimen. Examples of such include:

- Progress (Wyeth)
- Step-up (Cow & Gate)
- Forward (Milupa)
- Follow-on (Farleys).

The EU Scientific Committee for Food defines 'follow-on milks' as foodstuffs
intended for nutritional use in infants aged over four months. However, they are
not recommended in the UK until beyond six months of age.

These preparations contain more iron and vitamin D and less saturated fatty
acids than whole cow's milk. The great advantage of these formulations, which is
also true of standard infant formulas, is that if an adequate volume (500 ml/day)
is consumed, then the iron content will prevent the specific anaemia associated
with poor weaning diets. Doorstep cow's milk has only a fraction (one twenty-
fifth) of the iron content found in 'Progress' milk. Also, there is 60 times more
vitamin D in 'Progress' than in cow's milk, therefore reducing the likelihood of
rickets developing in a child who is receiving a follow-on milk. The amount of
calories is no greater than that found in other milks, and so obesity will no more
readily arise, given the daily intake is not excessive. These formulas are particularly useful in the 'faddy eater', where 500 ml/day will provide most of the
micronutrients and are suitable for use until the infant is two years old.

Soy-based infant formula

Soy formulas adapted for use in infants are derived from a soy protein isolate
and not the whole bean. They contain the approved amount of protein, fat,
carbohydrate, minerals and vitamins. Nevertheless, breast and cow's milk formulas
are the preferred sources of nutrition for infants (Department of Health, 1996).

Although having an odd odour and taste, soy formulas are free from cow's milk
and therefore may be suitable for some infants requiring a cow's-milk-free diet.
However, the use of soy-based formulas is associated with hazards.

- They contain relatively high concentrations of phytoestrogens.
- There is a high risk of developing an allergy to soy proteins – 15%–40% of
  children with cow's-milk-protein intolerance will also develop soy protein
  intolerance.
- Infants fed soy milk or soy formula may be at increased risk for subsequent
  peanut allergy (Lack et al, 2003).

In a report published in 2003, the Committee on Toxicology of Chemicals in Food
(COT) recommended that, owing to their high phytoestrogen level, soy-based
infant formulas be fed to infants only when indicated clinically (see p. 37). Furthermore, they are not recommended in infants under six months of age.

The concentration of phytoestrogens found in soy-based infant formula is several orders of magnitude higher than that in breast milk. A large body of evidence

documents the role of phytoestrogens in influencing hormone-dependent states. Infants fed soy formula receive high levels of phytoestrogens, in the form of soy isoflavones, during a stage of development at which permanent effects on their reproductive health are theoretically possible.

- In a retrospective cohort study conducted among adults aged 20–34 years, women who, as infants, had been fed soy formula reported a longer duration of menstrual bleeding and greater discomfort with menstruation compared with those who had been fed cow's milk formula (Strom et al, 2001).
- A study conducted in male neonatal marmosets found that feeding of human infant soy milk formula was associated with a significant increase in the number of Leydig cells in the testes and suppression of testosterone levels (Sharpe et al, 2002).

Where a doctor recommends soy milk, a complete baby-type of feed should be used, i.e. we support the appropriate and proper use of products such as SMA Wysoy (Wyeth), Infasoy (Cow & Gate) and Prosobee (Mead Johnson) as opposed to the incomplete adult preparations. The latter, although suitable as an adult drink, must not be offered to babies or infants because of their nutritional deficiencies: namely, the low mineral and vitamin content, as well as the wrong form of protein.

A hazard for mothers shopping in healthfood shops is that they might choose an adult type of soy milk for a child. Too many mothers are making ill-advised dietetic decisions regarding the merit of soy milk versus cow's milk. There is no irrefutable medical evidence that the use of soy milk will prevent the development of eczema, asthma, hayfever or other allergic disorders if given early in the newborn period. Casual use of soy infant formula in response to vague symptoms may delay diagnosis of underlying disease.

Care must be taken to prevent dental caries with soy and other lactose-free milks (this includes most therapeutic formulas), as the carbohydrate source is not lactose and therefore is more cariogenic. A history of early caries in both parents might imply a genetic predisposition as an additional risk factor in such an infant.

To minimise dental caries the following should be observed: soy milk or any therapeutic formula should be fed from a cup as soon as possible, and a feeding bottle should never be left with the infant overnight. Teeth should of course be brushed frequently.

Therapeutic infant formulas

These should only be used when medically indicated and always in conjunction with an appropriate diet. All such children must be under the care of a state registered dietician (SRD).

Hydrolysed cow's milk protein formulas

- Pregestimil/Nutramigen (Mead Johnson)
- Pepti Junior (Cow & Gate)
- Alfaré (Nestlé)
- Peptide 0–2 (SHS)
- Nan HA (Nestlé).

The protein in these formulas is hydrolysed so that they are hypoallergenic. They are the first-choice formulas in cow milk protein intolerance. They are also suitable for malabsorption syndromes and are prescriptible on FP 10.

Elemental formulas

- Neocate (SHS).

This formula is produced from synthetic amino acids. It is used in severe malabsorption and food allergy. It is prescriptible on FP 10 and is expensive.

Thickened formulas

- Enfamil AR (Mead Johnson)
- SMA Staydown (Wyeth).

These are nutritionally complete, casein-dominant formulas thickened with corn-starch. They are used for mild gastro-oesophageal reflux and are an alternative to adding a thickening agent to regular formula.

Novel formulas

- Omneo Comfort (Cow & Gate).

This is not prescriptible and is marketed for non-specific minor digestive disorders (e.g. colic, presence of hard stools, and posseting). There is little scientific data at present to justify recommending this formula.

Nanny goat formula

This is not prescriptible and is not widely used. Proteins in goat's milk (and, indeed, in soy milk) may cross-react with cow's-milk proteins; thus, goat's milk is often not a suitable alternative in cow's milk protein intolerance. Some cases of eczema do respond to goat's milk.

High-calorie infant formulas

- SMA High Energy (Wyeth)
- Infatrini (Nutricia).

The composition of these is listed in Table 2.3. They can be prescribed on FP 10 forms for disease-related malnutrition, malabsorption and growth failure, as advised by an SRD or doctor.

Table 2.3 Composition of high nutrient density feeds (per 100 ml product). From Bentley D, Lifschitz C and Lawson M (2002) *Pediatric Gastroenterology and Clinical Nutrition*. Remedica Publishing, London.

Product	Protein	Fat	Carbohydrate	Energy	
	(g)	(g)	(g)	(kcal)	(kJ)
Infatrini	2.6	5.4	10.4	100	419
SMA High Energy	2.0	4.9	9.8	91	382

Product	Na		K		Fe		Ca	
	(mmol)	(mg)	(mmol)	(mg)	(μmol)	(mg)	(mmol)	(mg)
Infatrini	1.00	23.0	2.60	101.4	13.39	0.75	2.00	80
SMA High Energy	0.95	22.0	2.25	88.0	19.64	1.10	1.42	57

Lactose-free formulas

• Enfamil LF (Mead Johnson)
• SMA Lactose Free (Wyeth).

These are marketed for treatment of temporary (transient) lactose intolerance following gastrointestinal disease. Any small-bowel enteropathy (milk protein intolerance, giardiasis, etc.) causing damage to the villi will temporarily deplete the bowel of lactase and other brush-border enzymes.

Soy-milk formulas

• Infasoy (Cow & Gate)
• Ostersoy (Farley's)
• SMA Wysoy (Wyeth)
• Prosobee (Mead Johnson)
• Isomil (Abbott).

These formula are high in phyoestrogens (*see* p. 45); therefore, it is recommended that they be used only when clinically indicated (COT, 2003). They can be prescribed on FP10 forms for proven lactose intolerance or cow's-milk-protein intolerance. They are not recommended in infants under six months of age. Their use may be justified in an older child with intolerance to cow's milk proteins who refuses extensively hydrolysed/elemental formulas, or in the rare infant with galactosaemia. However, in view of current knowledge, parents should be counselled regarding the potential adverse effects of soy milk. A link with hypothyroidism, autoimmune thyroid disease and an apparent increase in hypospadias might deter the carers from using this option.

All of the aforementioned specialised products, except the high-energy formulas, have a similar energy density (65–70 kcal per 100 ml) and protein content (1.4–2.0 g per 100 ml) and conform with UK and European Commission Directive guidelines.

Marketing of infant formula feeds

Breastfeeding advocacy must be maintained and monitored by governments (Waterston & Tumwine, 2003). It is important, for example, that formula manufacturers do not use the risk of maternal transmission of HIV infection as a pretext to encourage mothers to abandon breastfeeding. Distribution of free milk powder has been used by some producers of infant formula feeds – this is an irresponsible, unethical and potentially hazardous practice.

The International Code of Marketing of Breast Milk Substitutes (WHO/UNICEF, 1981) makes a number of recommendations.

- There should be no advertising of breast-milk substitutes to the public.
- No free samples should be given to mothers.
- There should be no promotion of products in healthcare facilities.
- No company nurses should advise mothers.
- No gifts or personal samples should be given to healthcare workers.
- No words or pictures idealising artificial feeding, including pictures of infants, should be on the labels of the products.
- Information to health workers should be scientific and factual.
- All information on artificial feeding, including the labels, should explain the benefits of breastfeeding, and the costs and hazards associated with artificial feeding.
- Unsuitable products, such as condensed milk, should not be promoted for babies.
- All products should be of a high quality and take account of the climatic and storage conditions of the country where they are used.

Unfortunately, many formula manufacturers fail to adhere to the Code. Furthermore, in a number of developing societies, there is little or no awareness amongst health workers of the Code.

There are a number of international bodies responsible for monitoring breaches of the Code: the WHO Common Review and Evaluation Framework, the International Baby Food Action Network (IBFAN), and the Interagency Group on Breastfeeding Monitoring (IGBM).

Preparation and storage of bottle feeds

All mothers who intend to bottle-feed should be shown how to make up feeds before discharge from the maternity unit.

Hygiene

A high standard of hygiene must be maintained when making up and storing feeds. One of the important potential hazards of bottle-feeding is that of bowel infections (gastroenteritis). This is upsetting for both the child and the parents and can, on rare occasions, be dangerous and associated with many complications. It is therefore of utmost importance that a clean and careful routine is observed at all times in relation to the baby's feeding materials.

The preparer must both wash his or her hands thoroughly and, more importantly, ensure they are properly dried before handling the powder and equipment for a feed.

Water is the main source of microbiological hazard in infant milk feeds. All water used for feeds or drinks for infants less than six months of age should be boiled and cooled before use. This includes bottled water (which is not sterile) and filtered water (water filters are a breeding ground for bacteria).

Types of water

As mentioned above, all water used for feeds or drinks for infants below the age of six months should be boiled and cooled before use. In some developing countries (e.g. Libya), boiled water contains too high a content of salt and other minerals, but this is not so in the UK. The recommended upper limit for sodium in a prepared infant milk is 35 mg/100 ml. Types of water **unsuitable** for making up feeds include:

• softened water – may contain an unacceptably high level of sodium
• repeatedly boiled water – contains a high level of sodium
• bottled water with added minerals
• natural mineral water – risks fluorosis
• sparkling bottled water – promotes wind and has a variable mineral content.

Measuring the feed

Feeds must be made to the correct strength and in accordance with the instructions on the packet or tin. In the UK, dilution is standardised to one level scoop of powder to 30 ml of cooled, boiled water. Mistakes in making up feeds are common and potentially hazardous: an overly concentrated feed puts excess stress on the baby's kidneys (particularly those who are immature), thus risking hypernatraemia (raised serum sodium), and can cause excessive weight gain.

Thus, the amount of powder used per measure of water must only be as directed, and scoops from different makes of powder must not be mixed. When measuring the powder, it must not be compressed into the scoop spoon. A sterile knife blade should be used to level off and so remove excess powder.

Storage and use

Feeds can be prepared in advance, then stored in sterilised bottles in a refrigerator and used over the next 24 hours. Storage for longer periods is unwise and so any unused bottles must be discarded. A cold feed ought to be warmed up and tested by the feeder against her or his own skin (traditionally the back of the hand). Milks only need to be heated sufficiently to remove the chill. Microwaves should not be used for this purpose, as they heat the milk unevenly and thus could easily scald a baby's mouth or even damage the oesophagus.

Technique of feeding

A wide variety of teats – both shape and material – are available. Some are modelled to fit the baby's palate and so allow control over the flow rate. The teat must be made with a hole that delivers the milk at a reasonable rate, namely a drop a second. It is important to remind mothers that thickened feeds, used for reflux, require a larger hole in the teat. If the hole is too small, flame a needle mounted to a cork to red heat and plunge it through the existing aperture to enlarge the diameter. However, too large a hole is risky, as the baby might choke when gulping the milk in big volumes.

Whilst feeding, it is necessary to pause at intervals, to allow air bubbles to collect on the surface of the milk within the bottle and so not be swallowed. As the bottle empties, a sufficient angle must be maintained for the milk to cover the whole teat hole; otherwise, the baby will swallow air and become distended, possibly leading to discomfort (Fig. 2.1).

An average bottle-feed may take 20–30 minutes, but there is no hard-and-fast rule. The baby's hunger and state of alertness will influence the time factor.

Any milk remaining after a feed should be thrown away and not re-used, as it could harbour bacteria, with the risk of introducing a bowel infection, even if stored in a refrigerator.

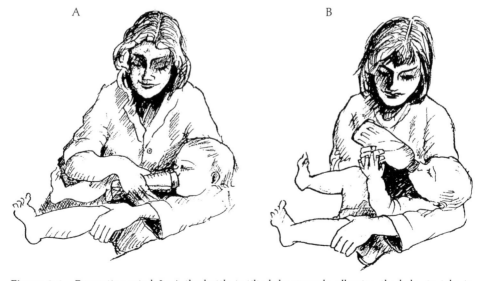

Figure 2.1 Preventing wind. In A the bottle is tilted downwards, allowing the baby to take in large quantities of air as well as milk. In B the mother is preventing wind by ensuring that the bottle is tilted to fill the teat with milk, so that the baby takes in only milk.

Babies should be formula fed on demand. However, as a guideline, the average daily volume for an infant (0–3 months) is 150 ml/kg body weight ($= 2\frac{1}{2}$ oz/lb). This calculation is based upon the actual weight, not the expected or projected weight (*see* Appendix 3 for further fluid requirements). If the baby fails to gain weight, the volume should be increased.

There are numerous reasons why a baby might cry when bottle-feeding, such as colic, etc. (*see* p. 20). A small hole in the teat results in slow feeding and perhaps a frustrated, if not an angry, hungry baby. When a baby is consistently unhappy on formula, fretful, snuffly, perhaps vomiting, especially if originally contented on human milk, then we need to consider cow's milk protein intolerance (*see* p. 96).

Sterilisation of bottles and equipment

Bottles, teats and storage containers can all be purchased, as can the products for sterilisation. There are a number of different ways to sterilise the bottles and equipment:

Sterilising unit

Instructions for setting up and using such units are set out in detail in the packages. These should be closely adhered to. It is important to remember that the tablets used for preparing the sterilisation fluids are dangerous if swallowed, and thus must be kept well away from inquisitive and mobile toddlers in the home.

To achieve adequate sterilisation, equipment must be soaked for at least three hours. Bottles and teats must be totally immersed, if not submerged, in the sterilising fluid, after being brushed to remove any milk curds or debris. This procedure is recommended right after a feed. Bottle and teat can then be stored, until needed, in a lidded plastic box containing the sterilising liquid. Neither the inside of a sterilised bottle nor any part of the teat should be touched unnecessarily. Teats – which, in Western Europe, are inexpensive – should be replaced in the storage solution if handled at the tip (where the hole is sited) or the inside (which will, of course, make contact with the milk). It is obviously important to remove the sterilising fluid from within a bottle and also the surface of the teat before a feed. Both can be rinsed with cooled boiled water.

Microwave sterilisers

These are specifically manufactured for the microwave. Teats and bottles are placed on a special tray and a specific quantity of water is added before the microwave is started. Sterilisation occurs via steaming, as below.

Steam sterilising unit

In this process, the bacteria are effectively and rapidly destroyed within a special piece of apparatus.

Dishwasher

Place the bottles and all the equipment (except the teat) into the dishwasher. The teat should be boiled separately.

Boiling

Bottle, teat, etc. are all boiled for 25 minutes in a large covered pot. Teats made of rubber will not survive too many boilings.

Different commercial forms of milk

Raw milk (from the cow, sheep or goat)

Raw milk must not be given to infants or children – nor, indeed, adults – and in a number of countries its sale is forbidden. Unfortunately, however, the sale of foods made from raw milk is not as yet forbidden within the European Union.

It is conceivable that a family isolated from shops or camping in a remote farming community might be tempted to try and acquire such milk from a local dairy farmer. However, this practice is extremely hazardous. Legislation exists to ensure such dairies are inspected periodically, to examine standards of hygiene and ensure milk preparation is of an acceptable measure – but these are not weekly inspections! Cattle must be free from tuberculosis (TB) and brucellosis. However, many harmful microbes apart from those causing TB and brucellosis – for example, *Campylobacter*, *Salmonella*, *Yersinia* and *Toxoplasma* species – can be traced back to the udder of the cow, sheep or goat.

Cow's milk

Pasteurised milk

The term 'pasteurisation' – derived from the work of Louis Pasteur, a French chemist – describes a process whereby milk (or other fluids, e.g. wine and beer) are heated to a high temperature and then cooled. The procedure kills most pathogenic organisms while retaining the flavour of the liquid. However, milk proteins will change (denature) as a result of the heat treatment. Nevertheless, we would recommend this type of milk, even though cow herds in the UK are said to be free of TB. It is essential to note that although the milk has been pasteurised by the dairy company it could, once unsealed – be it accidentally or deliberately, during manufacture, in transit, or at home – subsequently become contaminated, even if stored in a refrigerator.

In children over one year of age, a minimum of 300 ml of full-fat cow's milk, or the equivalent in dairy products, should be taken per day to ensure an adequate calcium intake. However, if more than 600 ml of full-fat cow's milk per day is consumed, it will deter feeding at mealtimes and could result in iron and other mineral deficiencies. Children can drink excessive volumes of milk.

Homogenised milk

Milk is an emulsion containing tiny fat droplets which, when the milk stands, will rise to the surface but will not coalesce. The purpose of homogenisation is to make the milk more digestible by breaking up fat globules. Post homogenisation, the composition of the milk is the same, but instead of containing fat globules with a large range of sizes (1–18 μm), there is a more uniform distribution of droplets with a narrow range in size (1–2 μm). Such modification will result in the milk looking uniformly whiter and having an evenly creamier taste.

This is suitable as the main drink for infants aged over one year. No more than 600 ml/day should be consumed, to avoid iron and micronutrient deficiencies.

Evaporated and condensed milks

Evaporated (unsweetened condensed) milk during production is heated and this procedure causes the loss of some of its water and a reduced final volume. The preparation contains no sugar and is sterilised. Evaporated milk is usually enriched with vitamins A and D. However, its exact composition is subject to the regulations in the country where it is marketed. Evaporated milk, if suitably diluted, can be used whenever cow's milk is appropriate, i.e. after 12 months of age.

Condensed milk is reduced to an even smaller volume by the heat treatment and is very sweet (owing to the high sucrose content). In the UK, it is a skimmed milk, and, if undiluted, has too much protein. Thus, here, this type of product is not suitable for adaptation into a feed for infants.

Sterilised milk

This variety of milk has been heated to boiling point and will keep indefinitely if the seal is intact and the bottle or carton is unopened. It has a distinctive flavour. In the very remote possibility of the germs that cause TB being present, they will not be destroyed in sterilised milk, in contrast to pasteurised milk.

UHT (ultra-high temperature) milk

UHT milk has been heat treated for one to two seconds at 138–158°C. Because of this process, UHT milk, which has an unusual taste, may be stored, unopened, at room temperature for up to three months from the date of processing. Because it does not need refrigeration, it may be useful for those travelling with children over one year of age. However, once opened, UHT milk must be used within four hours, or refrigerated in its original container and used within seven days.

Skimmed and semi-skimmed milk

Skimmed milk is most certainly not suitable for babies – or even infants under five years of age – owing to its low calorie content and deficiency in vitamins A and D. In some circumstances, such as obesity and hyperlipidaemias, however, it might be recommended. It is available as a powder or in ready-to-use liquid form. Skimmed milk has very little fat but contains almost all of the protein, lactose (milk sugar), minerals and water-soluble vitamins to be found in standard milk. It is an inexpensive by-product formed during the manufacture of butter. Dried skimmed milk plays an important role in food-aid to developing countries.

Semi-skimmed milk is not as deplete of fat as is the fully skimmed type, but it must not be used for babies or those less than two years of age. It can be given to children over two years of age if their diet is adequate in calories and vitamins A and D.

Goat's milk

There are many potential problems and disadvantages in using a milk which has evolved for the goat's kid and not the human species.

- Goat's milk is not subject to the same hygiene legislation as cow's milk and can be bought unpasteurised. Unpasteurised goat's milk is a potential source of many infections, including TB and brucellosis, which can be serious, life-threatening diseases. Dairy cow herds are closely monitored to ensure that they are free of TB and brucellosis (and other potentially dangerous infections that can be transmitted in milk). Furthermore, goats are usually hand-milked, which increases the chance of milk contamination by microbes from the skin of handlers. Although inspection and monitoring of dairy goats is developing, controls do not, as yet, embrace all herds. Voluntary guidelines have been laid down by the Goat Association.
- Goat's milk is not nutritionally complete: unless supplemented by the nanny dairy, it is insufficient in its folic acid content and so can cause a particular type of anaemia. Furthermore, levels of vitamins A, D, C and B_{12} are low.
- Goat's milk is richer in saturated fats than cow's milk and has a potentially high renal solute load.

Goat's milk must never be given to those under 12 months of age.

Carers of those who are allergic to cow's-milk proteins and suffering from eczema may use goat's milk in the hope that it will relieve the condition. The hazard is that, although the cow and goat are unrelated animals, their milks might have similar proteins and 'cross-react'; thus, a switch to goat's milk may not help.

If unpasteurised goat's milk is used, it must be boiled, even though this alters the flavour and lowers the micronutrient content, which is already reduced compared with cow's' milk − especially folic acid. It is now possible to buy goat's milk in powder form. However, health professionals rarely recommend it due to its similar allergenicity to cow's milk

Ewe's milk

Like goat's milk, ewe's milk is unsuitable for infants. The use of ewe's milk should be opposed for the same reasons as raw or unmodified goat's milk: it is nutritionally incomplete, has a high renal solute load, and may be microbiologically unsafe.

Also because of cross protein reactivity, ewe's milk and goat's milk can cause adverse problems in those with cow's milk protein intolerance.

Milk from other animals

Milk can be derived from a great many other domesticated herbivorous animals, including the buffalo, camel, reindeer, mare and ass. Although the greatest volume of milk in the UK comes from the cow, this is not so in India and parts of Africa, where it is obtained mainly from the buffalo. Different species produce milk of quite dissimilar protein, fat, sugar and energy content.

Soy milk

Unmodified soy milks sold for general use are unsuitable for infants under one year of age. They are likely to contain unmodified soy protein and may not include adequate minerals, particularly calcium (*see* also p. 37).

Further reading

- Lack G, Fox D, Northstone K *et al* (2003) Factors associated with the development of peanut allergy in childhood. *NEJM.* **348**: 977–85.
- Leung DYM, Sampson HA, Geha RS and Szefler SJ (2003) *Pediatric Allergy Principles and Practice.* Mosby, Missouri.
- Sharpe RM, Martin B, Morris K *et al* (2002) Infant feeding with soy formula milk: effects on the testis and on blood testosterone levels in marmoset monkeys during the period of neonatal testicular activity. *Hum Reprod.* **17**: 1692–703.
- Strom BL, Schinnar R, Ziegler EE *et al* (2001) Exposure to soy-based formula in infancy and endocrinological and reproductive outcomes in young adulthood. *JAMA.* **286**: 807–14.
- Waterston T and Tumwine J (2003) Monitoring the marketing of infant formula feeds. *BMJ.* **326**: 113–14.

CHAPTER 3

Preterm and low birthweight babies

Classification

Normal (term) birthweight is 3300–3500 g. Low birthweight (LBW) is a weight of less than 2500 g at birth and may arise in two groups of infants.

Box 3.1 Classification systems for describing infant size and age at birth.

Premature infant	An infant born before 37 weeks of gestation
Low birthweight	Birthweight <2500 g (5 lb 8 oz)
Very low birthweight	Birthweight <1500 g (3 lb 5oz)
Extremely low birthweight	Birthweight <1000 g (2 lb 3 oz)
Small for gestational age	Birth weight less than the 10th percentile for intrauterine growth
Appropriate for gestational age	Birth weight between 10th and 90th percentile for intrauterine growth
Large for gestational age	Birth weight greater than the 90th percentile for intrauterine growth

---

- Preterm (premature) births are those that occur before 37 completed weeks of gestation. Approximately two-thirds of LBW infants are born preterm and have a size appropriate for gestational age. The earlier a baby is born, the less developed the organs will be, the less it is likely to weigh, and the greater its risk for many problems.
- Small-for-date babies ('small for gestational age' or 'growth-restricted') may be full-term but are underweight. Their low birthweight results, at least partly, from slowing or temporary halting of growth in the womb. Approximately one-third of LBW infants are small for date.

The nutritional requirements and clinical management of these two groups are not identical. However, all LBW infants are at risk of nutritional inadequacy.

Preterm infants have:

- low nutrient stores, e.g. calcium, zinc, iron, phosphorous, vitamin A
- immature organ and enzyme systems
- high nutrient requirements.

Small-for-date babies have lower energy stores (fat and glycogen) than infants of normal birthweight, and are prone to hypoglycaemia. Nutrient requirements are high.

Feeding of premature and LBW infants
Early feeding

As a result of an immature suck–swallow–breathe pattern, preterm infants require some tube feeding until 35–37 weeks' gestation. The milk of choice is undoubtedly that of the mother.

Breast milk
Breast milk has the following advantages over preterm formula:

- improved feed tolerance
- reduced risk of sepsis
- long-term neurodevelopmental benefits
- lowered risk of necrotizing enterocolitis.

Mothers should be fully supported to express breast milk for their preterm babies. A hospital-quality electric breast pump will help in this regard. Such expressed breast milk (EBM) will not be of standard composition, as preterm mothers very appropriately produce richer milk for a couple of weeks post delivery. In fact, EBM is so important to the preterm infant that pasteurised banked donor milk would be the second choice of milk feed if it were freely available. Pasteurised milk retains some immunological advantages even though heat-labile vitamins, bile-salt-stimulated lipase and live cells are reduced or destroyed in the pasteurisation process.

When the infant is able to suckle, the mother should start breastfeeding to further encourage milk production.

Infants weighing less than 1500 g or those failing to thrive on 200 ml/kg/day of EBM will need additional nutrients in the form of multicomponent breast-milk fortifier, which should be added once the infant is tolerating full feeds.

Breast-milk fortifiers
Preterm infants fed human milk alone gain less weight and show slower growth rates than those fed on fortified human milk. Multicomponent fortifiers are recommended and several are available in the UK:

- Nutriprem Breast Milk Fortifier (Cow & Gate)
- SMA Breast Milk Fortifier (SMA Nutrition)
- Eoprotin (Milupa).

It is important to have clear guidelines on the neonatal unit for the use of breast-milk fortifiers as their addition to breast milk increases the risk of bacterial contamination. It also increases the osmolality of breast milk, which further increases with storage and warming, due to the enzymatic action on carbohydrates in the fortifier. There should therefore be limited storage of fortified milk and a minimum

Table 3.1 Composition of formulas designed for premature and low birthweight babies – the Tsang consensus recommendations and the European Society for Paediatric Gastroenterology and Nutrition Committee on Nutrition (ESPGAN-CON) recommendations. From Bentley D, Lifschitz C and Lawson M (2002) *Pediatric Gastroenterology and Clinical Nutrition.* Remedica Publishing, London.

Nutrient	Tsang/100 kcal Infant <1000 g	Tsang/100 kcal Infant ≥1000 g	ESPGAN/ 100 kcal	Comments
Protein g	3.0–3.16	2.5–3.0	2.25–3.10	Amino acid content of the protein should not be less than breast milk
Fat: Total g			4.4–6.0	Not more than 40% medium-chain triglycerides should contain monounsaturated fatty acids
Linoleic g	0.44–1.70	0.44–1.70	0.5–1.2	
Linolenic g	0.11–0.44	0.11–0.44	>0.055	
C18:2/C18:3	≥5	≥5	5–15	
Long-chain polyunsaturated fatty acids			Desirable additives	n–6 LCP 1–2% of total fatty acids n–3 LCP 0.5–1% of total fatty acids
Total Carbohydrate			7–14	Not more than 11 g/100 ml; acceptable carbohydrates are lactose, glucose, starch hydrolysates, and sucrose
Lactose g	3.16–9.5	3.16–9.8	3.2–12.0	Not more than 8 g/100 ml
Oligomers g	0–7.0	0–7.0		
Vitamin A μg	583–1250	583–1250	90–150	May be advisable to supplement 200–1000 μg/day
Vitamin D μg	125–333 Aim 400 IU/d	125–333 Aim 400 IU/d	not exceeding 3 μg	Cholecalciferol or ergocalciferol preferred; supplement to a total of 20–40 μg
Vitamin E μg	5–10	5–10	4–15	α-tocopherol:polyunsaturated fat ratio should be at least 0.9 mg/g

amount should be made up at any one time (ideally equivalent to one feed), avoiding having to discard this precious commodity.

Formulas designed for premature and LBW babies

LBW formulas are specific preparations suitable for babies in special care baby units (SCBUs). These ready-to-feed formulations contain water, maltodextrins, milk powder, fat, iron, vitamins and minerals, and are designed to meet the special needs of LBW infants (Table 3.1). During the last three months of pregnancy, foetal growth is almost double that of the full-term infant in the early months of life. Therefore, this rapid and optimal growth can be achieved by these particular modified cow's-milk feeds. Preterm infants have low stores of energy and immature absorption and digestive systems. Furthermore, the kidneys are less sophisticated than those of the term baby. The LBW formulas have been devised to fulfil these many complex needs.

Standard LBW formulas are for use in hospital only, usually until a weight of 2.0–2.5 kg is achieved. Nutrient-enriched post-discharge formulas (NEPDF) are available for preterm infants after discharge. They are generally reduced in nutrient density compared with formulas for hospitalised infants, though are still more nutrient dense than standard milks.

Post-discharge feeding

Preterm infants are often discharged at a weight of approximately 2 kg, significantly less than that of a healthy, term infant. Unless good catch-up is achieved, growth can remain retarded. It is vital that all LBW infants achieve good growth and catch-up growth in the first two years of life. The diet after discharge must provide adequate energy, protein and micronutrients to allow this to happen.

Following discharge, LBW infants may consume astonishingly large volumes of milk. If there is doubt about the mother's supply of breast milk, she should nurse every $1\frac{1}{2}$–2 hours during the day in the first 24–48 hours after the infant's discharge, to ensure adequate milk production. After this initial period, she should feed on demand; the infant normally feeds every two to three hours (8–10 feedings per day). Six to eight wet nappies per 24 hours indicate an adequate fluid intake. Milk should not be withheld for longer than four hours.

All mothers should be encouraged to breastfeed their infants, where possible, on demand; however, where this is not realistic, nutrient-enriched formulas prove a useful alternative to term formula. They have been designed to supply the nutrition required in smaller volumes of feed (preterm infants have been observed to consume up to 300 ml/kg/day of term formula post discharge). Data suggest that enriched formulas may improve growth, bone mineralisation and, possibly, neurodevelopment compared with term formulas (because they contain long-chain polyunsaturated fatty acids, whereas, until recently, term formulas did not). Some of these formulas also have the advantage of nullifying the need for separate iron and vitamin supplements post discharge. These post-discharge formulas are prescriptible up to the corrected age of six months. There are currently two NEPDFs approved by the Advisory Committee on Borderline Substances (ACBS):

- Nutriprem 2 (Cow & Gate)
- Premcare (Heinz/Farleys).

Solid foods

Traditional recommendations on weaning preterm infants have been replaced by more evidence-based practice to wean between four and seven months postnatal age. Weaning foods should be energy-dense to optimise the infant's growth. In practice, this may require adding oil or butter to cooked vegetables and double cream to puréed fruits. Introducing meats, fish and a variety of flavours early on in weaning is important to enlarge the infant's acceptance of foods. We have observed that preterm infants often 'do better' with food than milk and hence adequate weaning is vital. Marriott and colleagues studied a group of 68 preterm infants; half were weaned according to normal practice. Infants introduced to high nutrient-dense solids at an early age had better intakes of energy and protein at six months and better iron status and length growth velocity at 12 months corrected gestational age when compared with infants weaned according to normal practice.

Practical feeding strategies
- Introduce solids four to seven months from birth.
- Aim for energy- and protein-dense foods (70–105 kcal/100 g and protein range of at least 2.0–2.5 g/100 g).
- Increase nutrient density of foods by adding a little butter, vegetable oil, grated cheese or double cream.
- Progress quickly to puréed meat or vegetable and pulse mixes.
- Start finger foods by eight months.
- Introduce lumpy foods by nine months.
- Enlarge variety in taste and texture.
- Encourage self-feeding.
- Move onto family foods by 12 months.
- Continue breast or formula milk until one year of age.
- Follow-on formula is useful until the child is two years of age (because of extra micronutrients compared with cow's milk).
- Use vitamin drops until five years of age.
- Monitor for feeding difficulties – provide early intervention if needed.

Further reading

- Bradford N (2000) *Your Premature Baby*. Frances Lincoln, London.
- Lang S (2002) *Breastfeeding Special Care Babies*. Bailliere Tindall, Oxford.
- Marriott LD, Foote KD, Bishop JA *et al* (2003) Weaning preterm infants: a randomised controlled trial. *Arch Dis Child Fetal Neonatal Ed.* **88**: F302–7.

CHAPTER 4

Weaning

The term 'weaning' − derived from the Anglo-Saxon word *weian*, 'to accustom' − describes the process whereby the diet is expanded to include food and drinks other than breast milk or infant formula (Fig. 4.1).

There are many aspects of baby/infant nutrition in which the experts in dietetics and paediatrics disagree, but perhaps no subject is quite as controversial as weaning. The different opinions often reflect our ignorance, but we can give some guidelines to the mother, even though we must not be dogmatic about precise times of transition to solid food. Weaning begins when semi-solid food is given in addition to milk. Babies are conservative in their dietary tastes and prefer gentle changes rather than sudden alterations in diet; therefore, weaning should be a slow process, extending over a period of weeks, if not months. There is no merit in a rapid transition.

Age of weaning

When should you wean?

We believe weaning should be neither before four months ($17\frac{1}{2}$ weeks) of age nor later than six months (26 weeks). This matches the recommendation contained in the Committee on Medical Aspects of Food Policy (COMA) report 'Weaning

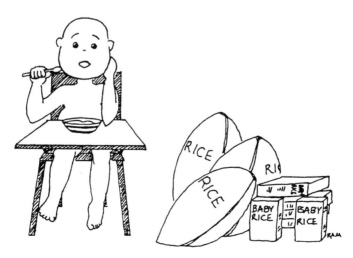

Figure 4.1   Weaning − 'to accustom'.

and the Weaning Diet ' (Department of Health, 1994). Current research supports the benefit of exclusive breast milk feeding until four to six months (Foote & Marriott, 2003), but there is a need for large randomized trials. However, to add some confusion to this already controversial topic, the World Health Organization (WHO) advises that infants be exclusively breastfed for the first six months, as it is deemed that breast milk provides all the nutrients most infants (i.e. healthy, full-term) need. The new UK Scientific Advisory Committee on Nutrition (SACN) has endorsed this WHO resolution, as has a recent (2003) statement issued by the Department of Health. Infants born before term by more than three weeks should be weaned somewhere between four and seven months or at six months if breast fed. We do not make such adjustments when deciding the age to begin immunisation procedures of preterm babies.

Why should babies not be weaned in the early weeks of life?

An important justification for delaying weaning until four to six months of age is that by then the bowel lining is more mature and sophisticated enough not to absorb foodstuffs that might cause allergic, or potentially allergic, reactions (*see* p. 3). Before the gut wall undergoes change with development, there is a greater chance of toxins being taken up (from foods or bacteria) and risk of subsequent illness.

Other physiological reasons to avoid early weaning include the excess demand that is put upon the infant kidneys due to the high renal solute load from foods. This is especially so if salty products are given. It has been suggested that the reduction in coeliac disease that has occurred in the past decade is linked to new habits of weaning. Coeliac disease is a disorder of the small bowel caused by an intolerance to gluten, the germ protein present in wheat and other cereals. It is an uncommon small-bowel disease in the UK and US (1 : 2000 children), but there is a high incidence in both south-west Ireland and central Italy. This disorder is serious but not dangerous in most circumstances. It is probable that the reduction in incidence of coeliac disease was occurring before weaning customs were altered, and is related to the later introduction of mixed feeds, the wider availability of gluten-free weaning foods (without any real justification), and the use of rice, rather than flour, as a first cereal

Also, there are developmental reasons why weaning should be delayed.

- Young infants have poor head control and cannot maintain an optimal position for swallowing unless aided.
- The ability to move food around the mouth and chew does not develop readily before three to four months.

Finally, nutritional reasons to delay weaning include the following.

- Breast milk can provide all the nutrients a baby needs until six months of age.
- Solids, given close to a breast feed, can reduce the absorption of nutrients (e.g. iron) from the milk.
- High-energy foods could cause early obesity.

Are there problems associated with very delayed weaning?

If weaning occurs much after six months, the infant is at risk of being deficient in iron, as well as energy, protein, and vitamins A and D. The term infant has a store of iron that will last until the birth weight has approximately doubled or until about six months of age. In the UK, all standard and specialised infant formulas are fortified with iron – that is why it is recommended that infant formula is continued until at least one year of age. In contrast, both breast milk and cow's milk ('doorstep' milk) are low in iron, the content being about one-tenth and one-twelfth, respectively, of that found in commonly used infant milks. Thus, babies given only breast milk or doorstep milk for prolonged periods have a higher chance of being deficient in iron. Those who use infant formulas or 'follow-on' milks in a quantity of more than 500 ml/day, or who are receiving iron, will not have this problem, but, as with all medications, iron should only be given if specifically prescribed. We are seeing too many babies in our hospital practices in East and West London with iron deficiency because of excessive and protracted use of doorstep milk and no exposure to solid foods containing iron. Introduction of cow's milk as the main source of milk before the age of one year, and the consumption of large volumes (> 600 ml/day) of such, are both risk factors for the early development of iron deficiency.

In addition, if weaning is delayed much beyond six months, difficulty arises because the infant will not readily adapt to new foods and methods of feeding. There appears to be a developmental 'window' during which it is easier to encourage an infant to taste a new food than it is at a later stage. Our London clinics are full of 'fussy' eaters, who will only accept yoghurt, bananas and custard, for example. This may in part be due to a lack of variety in weaning. Advice has changed from only introducing bland foods very slowly, to encouraging a variety of flavours in early weaning.

Another problem we frequently encounter is that caused by the delayed introduction of lumpy items – again, this leads to a significant reduction in dietary diversity. Lumpy and finger foods should have been taken by the age of eight months: a recent study by Northstone and colleagues showed that if such foods are introduced after 10 months of age, feeding difficulties are more likely to occur and children tend to have more definite likes and dislikes.

Strategy for weaning

The process of weaning can be commenced with one to two teaspoons of purée given at one feed per day when the infant is alert, before or during a breast- or bottle-feed. If the infant is overly tired or hungry, he or she may become upset and frustrated. Carers should attempt to introduce a new food daily, but there is no rule about how quickly weaning should occur, and much of the management is a matter of common sense. However, a variety of foods and flavours – particularly savoury – should be taken into the diet and may prevent faddiness at a later stage. Eggs and wheat should not be introduced before six months of age, but meat, fish and pulses should be tried by the first two months of weaning. Within two months, the baby should have increased his or her intake to three meals per day. Breast or formula milk should still be offered, but inevitably the volume will gradually decrease. A minimum of 500 ml/day of breast or formula milk is recommended until the infant is one year old.

The mother's attitude is important: a relaxed approach should be encouraged. Over the years we have seen many tearful mothers who, having spent much time and effort preparing the food, feel personally rejected when it is refused by their offspring. Sadly, mealtimes can become confrontational – this must be recognised and avoided. Even if speech has not yet developed, an infant will sense the mother's enthusiasm to ensure every teaspoon of her own food, prepared with great care and attention, is eaten. When a commercial food is refused, this seems emotionally less painful, presumably because the product has come from an impersonal retail source.

We must not underestimate the love and warmth which food-giving represents and, equally, the pain to the mother when it is spat out. The more the mother becomes stressed and emphatic about her baby consuming every mouthful, the greater the depth of feeling evoked in the infant.

Commercial preparations versus home-made foods

Both types of food have a place. Home-made foods are not always nutritionally sound but, because of variations in texture, best prepare an infant for later family foods. Commercially available weaning foods conform to strict compositional guidelines and are a great benefit to the busy mother who does not have time if working, or with a large family. In one UK study involving 5000 mothers, over 80% acknowledged that they used commercially prepared baby foods as opposed to their own home-made meals.

Commercial products

Ready-to-feed jars and tins of baby foods are made by Cow & Gate, Heinz, Boots, Milupa and Hipp Organic, etc. An alternative to the open-and-serve jar or tin is the dry powder in a packet, which needs added water or milk.

Mothers are presented with a great variety of choices when selecting foods for their babies. There would seem to be an ever-expanding programme by the manufacturers, who now market non-dinner baby meals, such as baby breakfasts, baby teas, baby snacks, baby suppers and soft drinks.

Commercial preparations are now very carefully labelled and are free of added sugar, salt and gluten, etc. This does not mean they are pure food products, however, because modern food-technological methods have been used in their creation and the manufacturer may have had to put in preservatives, colours, flavours, sweeteners, processing aids, 'stabilisers', 'antioxidants', and 'emulsifiers', etc. In the UK, only 26 additives are prohibited in baby foods. The use of additives is regulated in the UK by the Food Advisory Committee in the European Union by the Scientific Committee for Food.

Contamination

Jars have been contaminated by people menacing or commercially sabotaging a company's product and damaging the safety record as well as public confidence. Seals to jars have recently become more sophisticated to show the carers there is less risk of product interference before consumption. However, jars can have imperceptible or hairline cracks which allow bacterial entry. Tins do not pose such problems and strict laws exist regarding the hazards of contamination by heavy metals, particularly lead. In 2003, traces of the chemical semicarbazide (SEM) were identified in glass jars containing baby foods. The source of SEM is probably from the plastic sealing gasket used in the metal lids. The European Food Safety Authority (EFSA) Ad Hoc Expert Groups report concluded that SEM is present in certain foods in very low quantities. As yet it has not been exensively studied but the experts believe the health risk is very small.

In 1986, Heinz in America declared they would remove pesticide residues from their baby products, and Milupa, too, gave some assurances regarding their surveillance policy relating to such pollutants. Yet, unless the constituents are selected very carefully, a mother's own home-made dinners could similarly pose a potential risk. Nevertheless, mothers can be assured that home-made meals will not have unnecessary thickening materials (e.g. starch), or a high water content, which is often present to a considerable degree in many commercial baby foods.

Hygiene

Theoretically, one major benefit of manufactured versus home-made meals is that of hygiene. Handling of food by mothers whilst cooking can result in the introduction of microbes – the degree of this risk is influenced by the carer's level of education, skills and awareness of cleanliness, as well as the facilities available. Processing techniques used by manufacturers are such that it is rare, but not unknown, for their products to become contaminated by bacteria.

Parents and other carers need to be alerted to the potential hazards to food when pets are in the household. Organisms from cats, dogs, tortoises and indeed most pets (as well as farmyard animals) can all contaminate meals if children or adults are careless in the kitchen area and transfer, by hand, microbes to food or cooking utensils. This includes the water to be found within tropical fish tanks. Should a child's fingers become contaminated by handling the fish, or just the inside of the tank, he or she is at risk of Salmonellosis. Such rare cases have been described and indeed reported by the Public Health Laboratory Services at Colindale in London. Few children, especially toddlers, can resist touching their own lips if not fingers sometime after playing with a fish tank and its contents.

Food preservation
Storage of meals

Made-up baby meals should not be stored in a domestic refrigerator for more than 24 hours because of the risk posed if the food-container seal is not airtight. Bacteria can be introduced via many avenues. Opening and closing the door of a refrigerator will facilitate elevation of the temperature and also enhance the risk of contamination. Furthermore, many surveys have shown that, with age, domestic refrigerators often do not function efficiently and will not reach as low a temperature as they did when new. If the carers are prudent, they should heat all meals to a high temperature, especially meats and poultry. If there is ever any doubt regarding the safeness of the baby meal, it should be discarded.

Freezing

Freezing is the best method for long-term food preservation. Such food will retain most of its original flavour, colour and nutritive value. However, freezing can produce some deterioration of the food textures as a result of ice formation; fast-freezing minimises this problem. Preservation by freezing is achieved by lowering the temperature to at least $-18°C$. At this sub-zero level, microbes will not grow.

'Good eating habits' – or 'getting it right'

Although what constitutes 'good eating habits' cannot be precisely defined, there is a consensus view from various expert bodies. The following are pointers and not absolute rules that must always be adhered to.

- Milk – during the first 12 months of life, the milk that is given in normal circumstances should be either breast milk or an approved infant formula. Full-fat cow's milk can be used, undiluted, in cooking from four months of age, but should not be the major source of milk until the infant is at least one year. In children over one year of age, a minimum of 300 ml of full-fat cow's milk, or the equivalent in dairy products, should be taken per day to ensure an adequate calcium intake. However, if more than 600 ml of such is consumed per day, it will deter feeding at mealtimes and could result in iron and other mineral deficiencies. Semi-skimmed milk should be used only in those over two years of age; fully skimmed milk is unsuitable before the age of five years. If milk causes problems, a dietitian or paediatrician might suggest an approved infant soy milk. In the year 2000, soy infant formula was the sole food of more than 6000 British babies. However, in a report published in 2003, the Committee on Toxicology of Chemicals in Food (COT) recommended that, owing to their high phytoestrogen level, soy-based formulas be fed to infants only when indicated clinically and should not be used in infants under six months of age (*see* Chapter 2). The phytoestrogens can cause hypothyroidism and autoimmune thyroid disease. There is said to be a fivefold increase in hypospadias in the male offspring of vegetarian mothers, which some attribute to the hormone content in soy milk. Furthermore, soy milk is rich in aluminium. Also, because of cross-reactivity between proteins in cow, soy, ass and goat milk, switching to other sources might not be the solution to the problem. In the older child, parents should be made aware of the oestrogen content of soy milk and its unknown effects. A hydrolysed formula is definitely preferable to a soy option in many circumstances.
- Cereals or thickeners should not be put into feeding bottles unless a dietitian has so advised for a specific reason (e.g. a baby who refluxes).

- Salt should not be added to a baby's food, neither should sugar.
- Vitamins – although a well-balanced diet will supply daily vitamin needs, vitamin drops are recommended, preferably until the age of five years, for all children unless they are consuming over 500 ml per day of infant formula.
- An adequate mixed diet should include milk, meat, poultry, fish, pulses, cheese, fruits, vegetables, bread and cereals.
- Snacks – if needed to provide adequate calories, then crackers, fruit, bread and sandwiches are better options than sugary and fatty snacks.
- Nuts are better avoided in those under five years of age, as there is the risk of tracheal obstruction.
- Groundnuts (Arachis hypogea) and all nut products should be avoided in children under three years with a family history of atopy. Peanut allergy is also associated with the use of creams containing peanut oil, and, possibly, the use of soy milk as well as soy-based formula. Few practitioners are aware that ground-nuts (peanuts) are rich in arachis oil and that is present in many skin preparations. Abidec vitamin drops also contain this oil.

Sugar

As current commercial food preparations are free of sugar, it would seem appropriate for mothers, when preparing their own baby foods, also not to include sugar.

- A high intake of sugars is associated with an increased risk of tooth decay.
- Adding sugar seems to encourage a preference for sweet foods, which can contribute to excessive weight gain and may cause rejection of nutritious savoury foods later.

Salt

The newborn can excrete an excess of sodium chloride if given sufficient water, but, since at this time the concentrating power of the kidney is suboptimal, more water has to be given in proportion to the salt. A baby's renal function takes several months to reach normal efficiency. This is why weaning diets need to have a low salt content; otherwise, the baby retains relatively more salt than water and the extracellular fluids become not only expanded in volume but also hypertonic, with the risk of metabolic problems.

Parents are also often concerned about the potential medical risks in adulthood of a high salt intake in infancy. We suspect that their fears are linked to the relationship in adults between salt and an elevated blood pressure in those with known hypertension. In healthy babies over one year of age – and, indeed, children – there is no convincing evidence that we need be too concerned about normal salt intakes. A reasonable compromise would be to add just a little salt when cooking, if this is the family custom, but not to add salt at the table. Analogous to the situation with sugar, a good case can be made that if the palate does not become familiar with salt, then it is probable, yet not impossible, that children will not, when adults, want to consume large and unhealthy amounts of salt.

Table 4.1 Sodium content of foods.

High-sodium foods	Moderate-sodium foods	Low-sodium foods
Canned savoury pasta and rice dishes	Ordinary breads, breakfast cereals, biscuits, cakes, pastries, crispbreads	Plain flours, dietetic low-salt bread, rice, pasta
Canned, smoked, dried and fermented meat and fish; sausages, 'cold cuts', savoury spreads, meat extracts	Shellfish	Fresh meat, poultry, offal/organ meats, fish
Cheeses	Cow's milk and milk products, fermented milks and yoghurts, salted butter and margarines	Whey-dominant infant formulas, unsalted butter, double cream
	Eggs	
Canned in brine, dried and fermented vegetables and pulses; olives, pickles, tomato juice	Dried fruit, vegetables (cooked in salted water)	Fresh and frozen vegetables (cooked without salt); pulses; fresh, frozen and canned fruit and fruit juice, tomato juice (no salt added)
Canned and packet soups		
Savoury 'nibbles', crisps, salted nuts		Nuts
Sauces, ketchup, relish, salad dressing, food additives, flavour enhancers, stock and gravy makers, yeast extract, Vegemite, Marmite		Lard, cooking and salad oils, yeast, herbs, spices, pepper, vinegar
	Golden syrup, treacle, chocolate-filled sweets and candies	Sugar, jam, jelly, clear sweets or candies, ice lollies or popsicles
Baking aids, baking powder, bicarbonate of soda, baking soda		Salt substitutes (contain potassium or ammonium salts)
	Fruit cordials, instant tea and coffee, malted milk, fizzy drinks, mineral water, drinking water (depends on area)	Cocoa powder, tea, coffee, distilled water

It has been suggested that there may be particular infants with a genetic predisposition to the development of hypertension as a result of the body's over-reaction to the presence of dietary salt; fortunately, this association is not seen in the majority of children.

There are compositional guidelines for infant formulas and follow-on milks in respect of their concentration of salt. COMA (1994) recommended 'moderation' in the intake of salt. The report commented upon the high salt intake commonly consumed in the UK and questioned the advantage of a reduction. A sudden change from the low sodium (salt) intake of babies fed human milk or infant formula to the high salt content of some mixed diets is not a desirable transition. The experts recommend that parents aim at moderation in the amount of salt offered to children (*see* Table 4.1).

Foods containing high levels of salt (e.g. stock cubes) should not be used until the infant is over one year of age.

Iron

Foods contain iron in one of two forms:

- haem iron – found in meat, poultry and fish
- non-haem iron – found in green vegetables, cereals and nuts.

Haem iron is relatively well absorbed from the gastrointestinal tract (25%), whereas non-haem iron is poorly absorbed (5%–10%). Enhancers of non-haem iron absorption include meat and vitamin C (ascorbic acid); inhibitors include tannin (in tea), soy, dietary fibre, phytates (found in unrefined cereals and bread) and phosphates (present in milk, eggs and some plant foods). Iron absorption is dependent on iron status: low iron stores or elevated formation of red blood cells (erythropoiesis) will increase the percentage of iron absorbed from the diet.

Iron deficiency can result in:

- recurrent infections
- retarded psychomotor and cognitive development
- anaemia (*see* Chapter 8).

Due to the high national prevalence of iron-deficiency anaemia (*see* Chapter 8), good sources of iron should be introduced into the diet from four months of age: mothers can offer puréed liver, red meat, pulses, beans, green vegetables and iron-fortified cereals. Because iron stores become depleted around six months of age, it is important to ensure the infant becomes accustomed to these high-iron sources early on.

Hard-boiled eggs are another source of iron and are less sensitising than soft-cooked eggs: however, eggs should not be introduced before six months of age, particularly if there is a family history of food intolerance or allergy (*see* below).

Iron is found in infant formula and also in so-called follow-on milks. There is not much iron in doorstep milk (about one-twelfth of that in baby formulae) or in breast milk. However, in human milk, the reduced content is compensated for by it being more readily available to the baby (i.e. it is of greater 'bioavailability').

The sources and functions of iron and other trace elements are listed in Table 4.2.

Table 4.2 Trace elements – sources and functions. From Bentley D, Lifschitz C and Lawson M (2002) *Pediatric Gastroenterology and Clinical Nutrition*. Remedica Publishing, London.

Name	Functions	Dietary sources
Iron	Haemoglobin and myoglobin; part of some enzyme systems	Liver and red meats, wholegrain cereals, fortified breakfast cereals, pulses (poorly absorbed from egg and dark-green vegetables)
Zinc	Part of >200 enzymes; involved in most areas of metabolism	Shellfish, meat, wholegrain cereals, nuts
Copper	Part of several enzymes – energy transfer and collagen synthesis	Green vegetables, fish and shellfish, liver, pulses, nuts
Selenium	Part of several enzymes – thyroid function; antioxidant	Wholegrain cereals, liver, meat, fish
Iodine	Part of thyroid hormones – metabolism and integrity of connective tissue	Fish and shellfish, meat, eggs, milk, vegetables
Chromium	Potentiates insulin action; involved in cholesterol metabolism	Yeast, beer, egg yolk, wholegrain cereals
Manganese	Part of several enzymes – glycolysis, polysaccharide synthesis	Tea, pulses, nuts, wholegrain cereals
Molybdenum	Part of several enzymes – uric acid metabolism, iron metabolism and sulfur metabolism	Wholegrain cereals, pulses, vegetables

Allergenicity

Infants are most vulnerable to the initiation of food allergy in the first months of life. It is prudent – particularly if there is a strong family history of atopic disease such as eczema and asthma – to withhold egg, egg products, wheat, milk and milk products (if solely breastfed before) until after the age of six months. However, such measures cannot guarantee that allergy will not appear, although some investigators have shown this policy has reduced the incidence of eczema in those who are predisposed. There is evidence to show that probiotics such as Lactobacillus GG capsules (lactobacillus rhamnosus) given antenatally and post-delivery will reduce atopic eczema in the breastfed.

Dietary fibre (non-starch polysaccharide/NSP)

Dietary fibre consists of several different components derived from the indigestible parts of plants and can be divided into two groups:

- soluble fibre (mostly gums and hemicellulose) found in fruits and vegetables
- insoluble fibre (bran and cellulose) present chiefly in cereal foods.

Dietary fibre cannot be absorbed and passes straight along the inside of the bowel, binding with water and some nutrients during its passage. The two types of fibre are treated differently in the large bowel but both have a part to play in increasing stool bulk and softness as well as stimulating colonic peristalsis (Fig. 4.2).

There is a consensus opinion among nutritionists that fibre intake is inadequate in the UK. Foods such as dairy products, meats and refined foods which have had their fibre removed during processing are major constituents of the diet in Britain. A low dietary fibre (or roughage) intake has been potentially linked with a number of bowel disorders. Most certainly, an important aspect in the management of constipation in children is to ensure that there is adequate fibre in their diet. Other diseases which might be associated with fibre deficiency include diabetes mellitus, diverticulosis (seen in some adults) and, perhaps, colonic cancer.

Currently there are no UK recommendations on fibre intake in children, although the average amount is low at less than 5.8 g per day. However, fibre-rich diets are not recommended in infants because of their low energy content and high bulk value. The American Heart Foundation has suggested an intake of age plus 5 g per day if over two years. The American Academy of Pediatrics has advised 0.5 g/kg/day.

High-fibre foods (see Table 4.3) should be encouraged, particularly wholemeal bread and cereals. Children may refuse wholegrain bread because of its colour, but high-fibre white breads are now available. Although children are renowned for their dislike of vegetables, peas and baked beans, which are good sources of fibre, might be acceptable. Puréed vegetables can be added to soups or sauces, but are less effective than raw or lightly cooked foods because they are more easily degraded in the bowel.

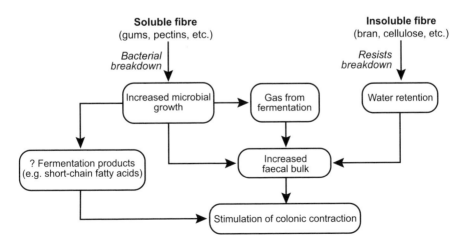

Figure 4.2   Action of dietary fibre. (Courtesy of Dr M Lawson.)

Table 4.3 Fibre content of foods. From Bentley D, Lifschitz C and Lawson M (2002) *Pediatric Gastroenterology and Clinical Nutrition.* Remedica Publishing, London.

Good fibre sources	Lesser fibre sources
Cereals	
Bran (wheat)	
Bread − wholemeal/wholewheat, brown	Bread − white
	Cornbread/tortilla
Chapatti − wholemeal	Chapatti − chapatti flour
Rice, boiled − wholegrain	Rice, boiled − white
Biscuits/cookies/crackers − wholegrain (e.g. 'Digestive', graham crackers)	Biscuits/cookies − white flour
Crispbread − rye	Crackers
Breakfast cereals − bran based, wholewheat, corn based, muesli type	Breakfast cereals − rice based
Fruits	
Berry fruits	Strawberries
Banana	Apple − raw
Dates − fresh	Grapes
Damsons − raw	Orange
Prunes − stewed	Mango
Raisins, sultanas	Melon
Nuts	
Peanuts	
Peanut butter	
Coconut − fresh	
Other nuts	
Vegetables	
Potatoes, boiled − old, new	Cucumber
Potato-crisps/chips	Lettuce
Root vegetables	Tomato
Leafy vegetables	
Spinach	
Beans − green, dried, boiled/refried, baked	
Peas, boiled	
Lentils, boiled − dhal	

It should not be necessary to add bran to a diet and there is some evidence that mineral balance is altered when bran is given as a supplement. However, in refractory constipation, if a child rejects a high-fibre diet, bran can be incorporated into home-baked cakes and biscuits and mixed with savoury gravies, sauces and soups. A coarse bran is preferable to a finely ground one. Large particles are less quickly degraded in the colon and have a better water-holding capacity.

Vitamins and weaning

Specialist advisory bodies such as the Nutrition Standing Committee of the Royal College of Paediatrics and Child Health advise vitamins A, C and D before and during weaning and preferably until the age of five years. Because it is not easy to determine on a day-to-day basis whether a weaning diet is sufficiently balanced to provide acceptable amounts of vitamin A, nor if sunlight exposure is adequate for vitamin D, supplementation until the age of five years is a recommended practice. We also need to remind vegetarians that vitamin B_{12} supplements will be required. Foods and drinks containing adequate sources of vitamin C and iron ought to be encouraged in the weaning regimen.

In a UK report published in 1994, the expert group COMA made the following recommendations.

- Breastfed infants under six months do not need vitamin supplementation, given the mother was not depleted of vitamin(s) in pregnancy.
- If an infant consumes 500 ml a day of either infant formula or follow-on milk, then vitamin supplements are not indicated until the infant stops taking formula.

Recent guidelines (2003) from the American Academy of Pediatrics have suggested that all infants have a minimum of 200 IU of vitamin D per day; supplementation is therefore recommended in all breastfed infants, to be commenced within the first two months of life. There has been a resurgence of rickets in the UK and this may have been exacerbated by fears of overexposure to the sun. Current recommendations suggest that infants under six months should not be exposed to direct sunlight. In addition, in certain cultures, the infant is covered excessively; so, we see a high prevalence of vitamin D deficiency in some UK Asian infants and others from vulnerable ethnic minority communities.

Department of Health vitamin drops are available from child health clinics. They are free to mothers and children who qualify for milk tokens. They contain 200 μg of vitamin A, 20 mg of vitamin C and 7 μg of vitamin D within the recommended five drops per day.

Day-to-day practice

By the age of nine to 12 months, children can manage many of the foods eaten by other members of the family. It is important the texture of the items offered are now more of a minced or chopped consistency. In clinic, we frequently see children who are still eating purées at 18 months of age or later. A feeding history often shows these children were introduced to lumpy foods too late. There appears to be a critical window of time between six and nine months when lumpy foods are more easily accepted into the diet. When we see children where this has

Table 4.4 Foods to be encouraged/discouraged.

Encourage	Discourage or limit
Vegetables	Fatty foods
Fruit	Sweets
Bread, pitta, chapati	Cakes, biscuits
Meat	Puddings
Fish	Sugary drinks
Poultry	
Potatoes	
Paste	
Rice	
Beans, peas	
Lentils, dahl	

not occurred, much more perseverance is required from the parents to ensure acceptance of different textures. Finger foods should be introduced gradually from six months of age. Examples of foods that should be encouraged, and those that should be discouraged or limited, are listed in Table 4.4.

What is a balanced diet?

Food from each of the following groups will enable a reasonable balance to be achieved (Fig. 4.3):

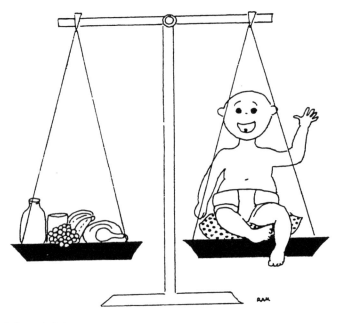

Figure 4.3 A balanced diet.

- Group 1: cereal foods, bread, chapati, pasta, rice, potatoes
- Group 2: fruits and vegetables
- Group 3: meats, fish, poultry, eggs, nuts, lentils and beans
- Group 4: milk, yoghurt, and cheese.

Foods from each group should be taken daily and those in Groups 1 and 2 need to be the basic source as well as two portions from Groups 3 and 4.

The best drinks for an infant are breast milk or formula, and water. It is important that infants are not given juices (even fresh) or squashes between meals as these will impede the infant's appetite and are bad for oral health. A child whose parents feel is not eating is usually drinking far too much. In our experience, infants often prefer to drink rather than eat, and the basic advice to improve intake is to offer only water or milk as a drink, and, in the infant over nine months, restrict formula/ breast milk to under 600 ml/day – usually offered in no more than three or four feeds in 24 hours.

How to encourage an infant/toddler to eat more

- Allow the infant to make a mess and explore his or her foods.
- Give infants more attention when they eat well and less when they refuse the food. A child may try to gain attention by refusing food, especially if he or she is unhappy or insecure. An infant can exercise considerable power within a family by rejecting food and causing parental distress. Mealtime must not be an opportunity for 'battle stations'.
- Children should never be force-fed. If the infant refuses to eat, the food should be taken away without comment. Unfortunately, in some cultures, force-feeding is acceptable. Parents should be informed that forcing children to eat is always a detrimental practice.
- Give food that they can hold themselves. This will help to develop co-ordination and acceptance of lumpy foods, as well as encourage an essential ability to chew.
- Offer a variety of foods – research shows that children need to try a new food perhaps as often as 14 times before it is accepted into their diets.
- If a child is to be encouraged to eat a bigger range, offer a choice of non-preferred foods so he or she maintains some control.
- Do not offer crisps and biscuits close to a meal.
- Make sure the child is not thirsty, as such an infant may eat less. However, carers should not fill up a child with drinks before meals. Remind parents that a thirsty child will drink water and that this is the best non-milk fluid.
- Do not hurry the child to eat, but, equally, mealtimes cannot become a continuing buffet.
- If problems persist the clinician needs to consider organic disorders, such as gastro-oesophageal reflux or dysmotility of the intestinal tract.

Vegetarian weaning

Of late in the UK, we appear to have witnessed a considerable vogue within many families of a commitment to a vegetarian regimen. In part this is due to the number of immigrants who follow a vegetarian diet, but, in addition to that, the indigenous population has become more enthused about the virtues of a meat/fish-free discipline. In principle, there are a number of obvious plus factors in such an approach to health; namely, vegetarianism usually involves a high fibre intake and a reduced consumption of cholesterol-containing foods. Moreover, the obvious good health of sensible vegetarians is propaganda in itself. Very restrictive vegetarian diets can pose problems to adults, but weanlings are at particular risk, because they need an adequate energy intake for growth. If a mother has had a suboptimal diet during pregnancy, then her breastfed infant will suffer the same deficiency disorders, especially in terms of vitamins and minerals. In the East End of London, we see a number of cases of rickets due to a vitamin-D-deficient mother producing vitamin-D-deficient milk.

Further reading

- Department of Health (1994) *Weaning and the Weaning Diet*. Report on Health and Social Subjects 45. HMSO, London.
- Foote KD and Marriott LD (2003) Weaning of infants. *Arch Dis Child*. **88**: 488–92.
- Hamlyn B, Brooder S, Lleinkova K *et al* (2002) *Infant Feeding Survey 2000*. The Stationary Office, London.
- Northstone K, Emmett P and Nethersole F (2001) The effect of age of introduction to lumpy solids on foods eaten and reported feeding difficulties at 6 and 15 months. *J Hum Nutr Diet*. **14**: 43–54.

CHAPTER 5

Vegetarian and other restricted types of diet

Types of vegetarian diets

The term 'vegetarian' is not a precise or specific one and there are many variations by those who adhere to such dietetic customs. Some followers abstain totally from all animal and fish foods, as well as eggs and dairy products of all descriptions. Others adopt amended regimens.

- **Semi-vegetarians** will eat no red meat but find fish and white meats (chicken, etc.) acceptable. However, the diet might be much more flexible than stated, and will vary from person to person, according to his or her own disciplines.
- **Lacto-ovo vegetarians** eat no meat, fish or poultry but accept dairy products and eggs. Yogic vegetarians are lacto-ovo vegetarians who will eat only natural and unprocessed foods/drinks.
- **Lacto-vegetarians** will eat dairy products and drink milk, but disapprove of animal foods.
- **Total vegetarians (vegans)** do not eat any animal foods (meat), dairy products or eggs. The vegan diet is likely to be implicated in serious disorders such as vitamin B_{12} deficiency and rickets, but vegans will accept B_{12} and vitamin D supplements. Although they ingest no dietary B_{12}, bacteria in the bowel will produce some of the deficient vitamin; thus, the problem is often theoretical, but can arise and cause major complications. Rickets is well described in vegan children. Some nutritionists claim that if a vegan diet contains a good mixture of cereals, pulses, nuts, fruit and vegetables with fortified soy milk or B_{12}, calcium and vitamin D supplements, the diet is adequate. However, it is essential that the diet is not low fat; indeed, extra oils often need to be added to ensure sufficient calories. Past research has shown that vegan children are shorter and lighter than their non-vegan counterparts.

It is apparent that a dietitian must be closely involved in advising parents who follow a vegetarian diet. Furthermore, the importance of an expert in dietetics is more critical in the case of veganism.

   Fruitarians only tolerate fruits, nuts and seeds (usually eaten uncooked) and exclude cereals and pulses as well as animal foods. Clearly, such a restricted diet is dangerous for a child and could involve doctors/social workers applying for court supervision to remove the child from the parents on the grounds of nutritional maltreatment. These potential hazards are similarly faced by infants offered a restrictive type of macrobiotic regimen.

One important observation we wish to make is that we have noted in families from the Indian subcontinent that very often mothers will be strict adherents to a vegetarian regimen of varying limitations, but will exclude their children, especially the babies/infants, from following their own dietary philosophy. The variation of adherence from mother (more so than father) to children is very considerable; therefore, dietary supplements must be based on the baby's dietary insufficiencies and not those of the parent.

Religious cultures and sects that follow dietary restrictions

Judaism

As within many religions, there is a spectrum of dietary restrictions practised, ranging from those adhered to by the ultra-orthodox down to the few dietetic restraints within some divisions of the religion. Those who are orthodox cannot eat fish unless scaled with fins – crustaceans must not be eaten (Deuteronomy 14: 9–10); nor pork products, nor meats unless the animal has split hooves and chews the cud and has been killed in a specific manner. Weanlings are not at risk because the diet is not that restrictive, although in some isolated communities, Kosher foods (i.e. prepared by an acceptable method) are not to be found, and mothers might then adhere to a lacto-ovo-vegetarian diet.

Hindus

The practice of non-violence against animals means that Hindus should eat neither animal meat nor fish, but restrictions do vary. No practising Hindu will eat meat from the cow or buffalo, as these are considered sacred animals, nor pork products, because the pig is deemed 'unclean'. Strict Hindus do not eat eggs or bulb vegetables (onions, garlic and leek). Milk and ghee (clarified butter) are regarded as sacred foods and are taken freely; thus, dairy products and pulses are important providers of otherwise excluded nutrients.

Jains

Jains are members of a non-Brahminical Hindu sect with dietary restrictions similar to Buddhists. They are strict vegetarians and often fast. Many avoid 'hot' foods such as eggs, fish, tea, honey, lentils, carrots, onions, ginger and chilli.

Islam

As with other religious faiths, some are strict adherents and others follow a less rigid regimen. Pork products and blood of all animals must be avoided. Animals must be slaughtered by the 'Halal' (unharmful) ritual. During Ramadan, followers must fast from sunrise to sunset, but young children are usually exempt from such a practice.

Sikhism

Their dietary customs are not dissimilar from those of Hindus, even though of a different faith. The diet is usually free of pork and beef. Meat when eaten must be from animals killed by 'jhatka'.

Buddhists

Strict adherents will not eat eggs, milk or any living animal that has been killed.

Seventh Day Adventists

These do not eat meat nor ingest stimulants (e.g. tea, coffee, chocolate, many food flavourings). Milk is allowed. Some Seventh Day Adventists are vegans.

Bahais

Many, but not all, followers are vegetarians. The ultimate goal is to reach a diet of fruit and grains only.

Rastafarians

Orthodox Rastafarians avoid all animal products, eggs, alcohol, salt and canned foods. Preserved foods are 'chemical' and to be avoided. Strict Rastafarian diets present problems for weanlings, and rickets has been described in the children of followers. Acceptable foods are 'total' (I-tal) or 'natural'.

Zen Macrobiotics

Zen Macrobiotics are described as followers of a 'nutritional system aiming to establish a healthy, happy life with spiritual awakening'. There are different dietary levels of this Taoist philosophy. With increasing stages, foods are withdrawn, so that finally the diet is most 'elemental and natural' (whole grains and liquids – but used sparingly). White sugar is avoided. Exotic foods are prominent. The single cereal diet (usually rice) with minimal fluid is proposed as the best food to achieve a state of wellbeing. Parents have been taken to court because of the deficiencies of such diets.

Hare Krishnas

These are lacto-vegetarians who stress natural and unprocessed foods.

From the aforementioned, it becomes apparent that some diets are so restrictive and limiting as to pose a hazard to a baby/infant (e.g. strict Zen-Macrobiotic diet, fruitarianism, etc.).

Food faddism is part of the child-abuse scenario. If a parent decides to offer his or her child a bizarre diet which is quite inadequate, then it must be made apparent to all that this is not acceptable, and falls within the huge spectrum of nutritional abuse.

Further reading

- Avery TM (1997) *Infant Feeding in Asian Families*. The Stationary Office, London.

CHAPTER 6

Vitamins

Vitamins are organic substances that occur in many foods in small amounts and that are necessary in trace quantities for the normal metabolic functioning of the body (Table 6.1).

In our experience, one of the most common questions that mothers are keen to rightly ask relates to that of vitamins. Perhaps this is associated with contemporary history and experiences of grandparents who sadly have seen deficiency-related disorders such as rickets, which even today is not that rare within UK Asian communities. Bow-legged children are uncommon within the indigenous population in Britain, yet many of us have witnessed this bone disorder in past decades.

Specialist advisory bodies such as the Nutrition Standing Committee of the Royal College of Paediatrics and Child Health advise supplementation of vitamins A, C and D before and during weaning and preferably until the age of five years.

Growing infants have specific needs if they are to maintain good vitamin status. In normal circumstances, it is uncommon to encounter clinical features of vitamin deficiency in British infants and children. Hopefully, this observation will reassure parents, who are increasingly aware of the need for a balanced and adequate diet. Fortunately, most weaning and infant foods that are marketed do contain added vitamins at levels which are approved and have been reviewed by responsible food manufacturers having to cope with the wishes of well-informed parents and various lobby groups.

It is important to emphasise that just as vitamin deficiencies may cause diseases such as rickets (vitamin D deficiency) and, in the past, scurvy (vitamin C deficiency), an excess of vitamin supplements, given by over-zealous parents who wish to avoid the risk of certain illnesses, can, in some instances, cause serious problems – for example, an excessive intake of vitamin D can lead to hypercalcaemia and renal damage. If parents follow guidelines issued by expert groups such as the Child Nutrition Panel of the DHSS Advisory Committee on Medical Aspects of Food Policy (COMA) in the UK, then problems ought not to develop.

Vitamins can be divided into two groups:

- fat-soluble – vitamins A, D, E and K
- water-soluble – vitamin B complex, vitamin C and folic acid.

Table 6.1 Vitamins – sources and functions. From Bentley D, Lifschitz C and Lawson M (2002) *Pediatric Gastroenterology and Clinical Nutrition.* Remedica Publishing, London.

Name	Functions	Dietary sources
Vitamin A	Growth, development and normal differentiation of tissue; β-carotene is an antioxidant Deficiency causes xerophthalmia	Dark-green vegetables, yellow fruit Retinol – liver, fish oils, milk, eggs
Vitamin D	Calcium absorption – bone health Deficiency causes rickets	Oily fish and eggs; added to margarine in some countries
Vitamin E	Protects lipid membranes from oxidation; antioxidant	Vegetable oils, eggs, butter, wholegrain cereals
Vitamin K	Normal blood clotting	Dark-green vegetables, liver
Thiamin (vitamin B_1)	Carbohydrate metabolism Deficiency causes beriberi	Wholegrain cereals, yeast, liver, pulses, nuts, meat
Riboflavin (vitamin B_2)	Oxidation–reduction reactions	Milk, liver, yeast, eggs
Niacin	Part of coenzymes NAD and NADP Deficiency causes pellagra	Liver, meat, fish yeast, peanuts, wholegrain cereals
Biotin	Involved in metabolism of fats, proteins and carbohydrates	Meat, fish, milk, eggs, wholegrain cereals
Pyridoxine (vitamin B_6)	Cofactor for enxymes involved in protein metabolism	Liver, wholegrain cereals, meat, fish, eggs, peanuts, bananas
Cobalamin (vitamin B_{12})	Works with folic acid in DNA synthesis and myelin formation Deficiency causes megaloblastic anemia	Liver, meat, fish, eggs, milk, milk products
Pantothenic acid	Part of coenzyme A, involved in energy release	Meat, fish, milk, eggs, wholegrain cereals, vegetables
Ascorbic acid (vitamin C)	Integrity of connective tissue; antioxidant Deficiency causes scurvy	Citrus fruit, berry fruits, green vegetables, potatoes
Folic acid (pteroylglutamic acid)	Synthesis of purines, pyrimidines and some amino acids Deficiency causes megaloblastic anemia	Liver, green vegetables, fruit, nuts, pulses, eggs

Fat-soluble vitamins
Vitamin A (retinols)

Substances with vitamin A activity comprise:

- retinol (or groups of substances with similar biological activity)
- provitamin A carotenoids, which can be converted to retinol in the human body.

In the period of weaning, milk and formula constitute the principal sources of vitamin A. Later on, the main supply is usually in the form of carotene from plant foods.

Deficiency of vitamin A can lead to keratinisation of the cornea, with resultant corneal opacity and blindness. Some historical facts are of interest in this regard.

- In the 1920s, infant formula lacking vitamin A caused night blindness.
- Carotene was given to Royal Air Force pilots in the Second World War in the belief it would help enhance night vision and adaptation to darkness.

Vitamin A deficiency is rarely seen in British children on a normal diet. However, this is not true in Asia, where vitamin A deficiency is commonly responsible for xerophthalmia and blindness. Those in the West have sufficient vitamin A such that even if on a diet free of this vitamin, their stores in the liver will suffice for one year.

Recommended dosage is 450 μg/day – 600 ml of formula will provide 480 μg.

Retinol is one of the few vitamins which in excessive amounts is harmful. The complication of overdosage was formerly described by Arctic explorers who ate the liver of polar bears, which is very rich in this vitamin, and, as a consequence, developed hypervitaminosis A. This source of nutrition is said to be astutely avoided by Eskimos. Food faddists are at risk of intoxication from carrots and pumpkins. Children on excess vitamin A can develop carotenaemia, which is characterised by yellow pigmentation of the skin, notably the face and palms.

In 1990, the Chief Medical Officer in the UK, Sir Donald Acheson, advised pregnant women of the hazard of excessive quantities of vitamin A, because of the danger – although it was described as 'negligible' – of causing birth defects in the foetus. They were warned of the risks posed by the use of vitamin A supplements and by eating liver. Liver can contain very high concentrations of this vitamin, and the amount in an average portion might equal 12 times the maximum daily dose recommended for pregnant women. However, it was subsequently stated that eating liver or liver pâté was not a potential problem for non-pregnant women or those women planning pregnancy, or for children or men.

Vitamin D (calciferols)

Vitamin D can be derived from the diet or formed by the irradiation of 7-dehydro-cholesterol in the skin due to the action of ultraviolet light (Fig. 6.1). Deficiency of vitamin D in the growing child leads to rickets.

Theoretically, dietary vitamin D is not required in infancy – given there is adequate exposure to sunlight, sufficient amounts of the vitamin will be formed in

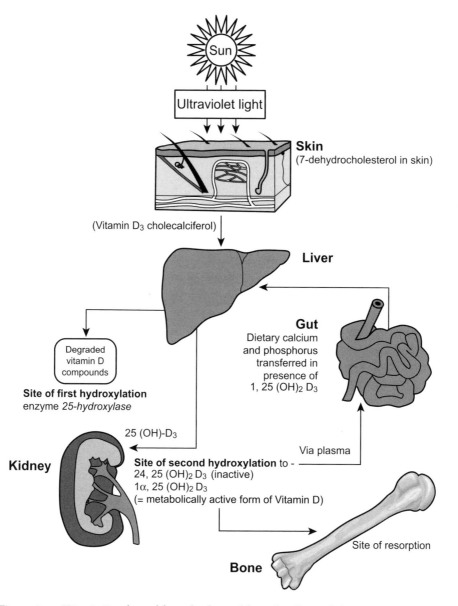

Figure 6.1 Vitamin D is derived from the diet and from the effects of ultraviolet light on the skin. It is hydroxylated in the liver to yield 25(OH)D$_3$ and undergoes a second hydroxylation in the kidney to produce the biologically active form, $1\alpha,25(OH)_2D_3$ (1,25-dihydroxycholecalciferol). $1\alpha,25(OH)_2D_3$ acts on the gut and bone to increase gut absorption and bone resorption. $24,25(OH)_2D_3 = $ 24,25-dihydroxycholecalciferol. (Courtesy of Professor P Byrne.)

the skin. Brian Wharton, Director-General of the British Nutrition Foundation, has suggested that the Clean Air Act in the UK might have played a role in improving the vitamin D status of mothers and their babies. Nevertheless, in many parts of Northern England, there is inadequate ultraviolet light because the smoggy, hazy atmosphere has prevented its transmission. The problem can be compounded by babies being swaddled or kept indoors, or even shielded within prams from light.

Also, mothers may remain within their homes in an endeavour to comply with the seclusion rules of the purdah system that is practised in some communities.

Inadequate sunshine may not be the complete explanation for vitamin D deficiency rickets, however, in that rickets was common in the 1940s in southern California and is today in India. The apparent rise in nutritional rickets that has occurred in American children of late (2001) may be due to a decrease in sun exposure coupled with a reduced use of vitamin-D-fortified foods.

If a mother herself is in a poor state of vitamin nutrition − e.g. has osteomalacia, which is an adult type form of rickets − then there is the potential hazard of her newborn developing rickets. Fortunately, some groups who are at particular risk have been identified from studies in Scotland and England, and there are guidelines suggesting that additional vitamin D − and, indeed, calcium − be given to Asian women in Britain who are pregnant. Mothers with extreme food fads and those consuming what have been described as 'exotic' diets put their children at risk.

Whereas human milk has a satisfactory vitamin D content (given the mother is adequately nourished and exposed to sunlight), cow's milk and many milk-containing foods are not naturally rich in their concentration of this vitamin. This observation probably accounts for the rarity of rickets in infants on breast milk. We must emphasise the need for vitamin D supplements in pregnant Asian women in the UK, as officially advised, and in both low birthweight babies (birth weight <2.5 kg) and children of Asian immigrants in the UK. This preventive measure will avoid rickets in the foetus and infant, and the disease of osteomalacia in an older child. In vulnerable infants, rickets might be noted when they switch from human milk to cow's milk. The reference nutrient intake for vitamin D is 7 μg per day in infants aged one to three years.

Most household diets are adequate in vitamins, except for D, which may or may not be sufficient. Current DHSS advice ('Present Day Practice in Infant Feeding: Third Report'. DHSS, 1988) suggests supplementation should be given from six months of age up to at least two years and preferably five years. In the COMA report 'Weaning and the Weaning Diet' (Department of Health, 1994), the panel of experts remind the reader of the toxicity of high intakes of D in all age groups, but infants especially are at risk. Timing of this supplementation should be influenced by such factors as the nature of the baby's milk (i.e. human or fortified), types of foods in the weaning diet (i.e. do they contain fortified milk, or, perhaps in contrast, have they been prepared by parents wanting to give an ovo-lacto-vegetarian diet?).

Vitamin E (tocopherols)

Vitamin E has a major role as an intracellular antioxidant, maintaining the stability of membranes, including those of red blood cells.

Low birthweight babies and those of less than 36 weeks' gestation are particularly susceptible to vitamin E deficiency. Placental transfer of tocopherol is low, and preterm infants are born with reduced stores.

There is a well-known association between vitamin E and reproduction in the female rat and between vitamin E deficiency and sterility in the male rat. This animal laboratory work has triggered the ill-justified use of vitamin E in well adults with fertility disorders.

Vitamin K (phylloquinone and menaquinone)

Vitamin K, a methylnaphthoquinone derivative, has a key role in maintaining normal blood-clotting mechanisms and preventing haemorrhagic disease of the newborn. If there is a deficit, intracranial bleeding can occur without warning, which can result in permanent disability and even death. In infants, intestinal bacteria are the main source of this vitamin, whereas in older children and adults, it is mostly derived from green plants. Breast milk is a poor source of vitamin K − although, of course, this does not deter us from discouraging formula feeding in babies. Because deficiency is potentially dangerous, it is the usual practice in maternity units to give vitamin K by mouth or injection to many, if not all, newborns. It is particularly relevant if forceps or a vacuum extractor is used.

A new vitamin controversy in 1992 was the alleged but unproven link between childhood cancers and injectable vitamin K. American paediatricians have not altered their practice because there is not, as yet, a licensed oral vitamin K product. In the UK, there have been official reminders of the need for vitamin K at birth, and ideally a second and third dose, especially in babies fed human milk.

Water-soluble vitamins

Vitamin B complex

This is made up of the following:

- Vitamin B_1 (thiamine) − this has an important role in preventing and curing the serious deficiency disorder beriberi. Beriberi is seen in South East Asia and is linked with the use of polished rice.
- Vitamin B_2 (riboflavin) − this has a major biochemical function; it is incorporated into flavoproteins and many enzyme systems.
- Vitamin B_3 (niacin) − deficiency causes a serious tropical skin disorder, pellagra.
- Vitamin B_5 (pantothenic acid) − this is a metabolic product of coenzyme A. Clinical deficiency syndrome has not been clearly defined.
- Vitamin B_6 (pyridoxine) − in the 1950s, a deficiency disease arose because a new baby formula had its pyridoxine content inadvertently destroyed during production. Convulsions can result from its absence.
- Vitamin B_{12} (cyanocobalamin) − this vitamin is one of the most important; deficiency will cause a serious type of anaemia (pernicious), as well as damage to the spinal cord. It is found only in foods from animal sources.

Vitamin C (ascorbic acid)

Vitamin C has a number of roles, including the capacity to act as a so-called 'antioxidant'. Also, it prevents scurvy, promotes wound healing, and can enhance iron absorption.

Historically, long sea voyages in the 16th and 17th centuries were associated with ascorbic acid deficiency because of poor nutrition. A vivid description of scurvy was given by Jacques Cartier in 1536, when his men were exploring the Saint Lawrence River:

'Some did lose all their strength, and could not stand on their feet ...
Others also had their skins spotted with spots of blood ... Their
mouths became stinking, their gums so rotten that all the flesh did fall
off, even to the roots of the teeth.'

A treatise by James Lind (1716–94), a British naval surgeon, documented that in a
controlled study in 1747, oranges and lemons could prevent scurvy, a disease
manifested by haemorrhages under the skin and within the joints, as well as
bleeding into the gums and often death.

It used to be though that water-soluble vitamins – such as vitamin C – in excess were harmless, in that they were either not absorbed or else excreted in the
urine. We now realise excess amounts can be hazardous. There is a dangerous
practice in which some parents give their children 'megadoses' to avoid upper
respiratory tract infections, etc. However, large doses of ascorbic acid are converted in the body to oxalates and excreted in the urine. Oxalate stones can be
formed in the kidneys and then found in the urine-collecting system. Although
there is some evidence to suggest that a generous intake of vitamin C will reduce
the incidence of some infections, it would be dietetically prudent to use a balance
of fruits and vegetables as sources.

The reference nutrient intake (RNI) is 25 mg/day for infants less than one year
and 30 mg/day in those over 12 months. Suitable nutrients (other than vitamin
preparations) comprise the juice of an orange, blackcurrant juice or rosehip syrup.

Vitamin C is destroyed by light, heat and oxidative processes such as cooking.
Cow's milk contains very little vitamin C, and pasteurisation and boiling of milk
reduces levels further. However, human milk is an adequate source of such; consequently, breastfed infants do not need vitamin C supplements.

Folic acid (pteroylglutamic acid)

Deficiency of folic acid (folate) is one of the most common vitamin disorders to
be seen in many populations. Body stores of folate at birth are small and can be
readily depleted as a result of growth, especially in small premature infants. The
folate content of raw goat's milk is much lower than that of human or cow's milk.
Infants fed on goat's milk without a folic acid supplement may develop megalo-
blastic anaemia. Although present in green vegetables, folate is easily destroyed
by excessive cooking, cooling and storage processes.

One of the most exciting pieces of research in respect of vitamins has been the
role of folic acid in the prevention of neural tube defects such as spina bifida.
The incidence of this serious spinal disorder could be reduced by 70% if all women
planning a pregnancy were to take a daily supplement of folic acid. However, the
supplement must be started pre-conceptually to be effective. Current UK government guidelines advise 0.4 mg/day be given for at least one month before con-
ception until the end of the first 12 weeks of pregnancy. However, a MORI survey
carried out in 2002 found that only 15% of women questioned took folic acid
before pregnancy. In view of such statistics, and because as many as half of preg-
nancies are unplanned, it is thought that pre-conceptual supplementation is imprac-
tical and that the only effective option is to fortify foods. However, fortification of
wheat flour and bread would not assist those in the Asian community who use

only chapati flour. This story is very reminiscent of the vitamin D saga and its subsequent problems in the proposed programme for the prevention of rickets within the UK Asian community.

The incidence of neural tube defects in the US has declined by almost 20% since the mandatory addition of folic acid to grain products such as breads, pasta, rice, flour and cereals in 1998.

There is some debate over the optimal level of fortification. The US adds 140 μg of folic acid per 100 g of grain. In the UK, a report published by COMA in 2000 called for fortification of all flour at a higher level – 240 μg per 100 g. It is said that this would reduce the risk of neural tube defects in babies by 41% without resulting in unacceptably high folic acid intakes for any group of the population.

Further reading

- Department of Health (1994) *Weaning and the Weaning Diet*. Report on Health and Social Subjects No. 45. HMSO, London.
- DHSS (1988) *Present Day Practice in Infant Feeding: Third Report*. Report on Health and Social Subjects No. 32. HMSO, London.

CHAPTER 7

Gastrointestinal disorders

Diarrhoea

Acute diarrhoea

At the end of the 19th century, the mortality caused by dehydration from diarrhoea worldwide was in the order of 80%. Now, in the US, within the population under the age of three years, the overall incidence of acute diarrhoea is about 1.3 episodes per child per year, but among children who attend daycare the rate is almost double. Diarrhoea accounts for approximately 9% of all hospitalisations of children under the age of five years, and almost 300 children die each year as a consequence of dehydration from diarrhoea (Fig. 7.1). Principally affected are premature infants, children of adolescent mothers, children of mothers who have received inadequate prenatal care, and children of mothers who are poor and/or belong to ethnic minority groups.

Most of the acute diarrhoeal episodes in children in the UK are caused by rotavirus. Breast milk is rich in antibodies to this infectious agent. Other common causative pathogens are the small round structured virus (SRSV) and adenovirus.

Management

The old concept of bowel rest has been completely abandoned for children with uncomplicated acute diarrhoea. Many studies have demonstrated that, once rehydrated, children with diarrhoea should receive their usual diet. At present, in well-nourished children in the developed world, carbohydrate malabsorption rarely follows rotavirus illness.

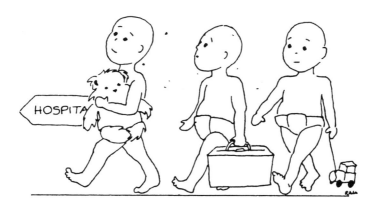

Figure 7.1   There are many hospital admissions because of gastroenteritis.

The treatment of choice to replace fluid and electrolyte losses is oral rehydration therapy (ORT). This can successfully rehydrate most infants and children at a lower cost and with fewer complications than intravenous therapy.

All kinds of beverages with a high carbohydrate content and electrolytes at non-physiological concentrations have been used inappropriately to treat children with diarrhoea. The use of such drinks can exacerbate the problem, as they have very low electrolyte concentrations and are hypertonic due to their high carbohydrate content.

Chronic diarrhoea

Diarrhoea lasting for more than 14 days is considered to be chronic.

The aetiology of chronic diarrhoea varies according to age. Common causes, *not* associated with growth faltering, include:

- excessive intake of fruit juices and high-carbohydrate beverages
- chronic non-specific diarrhoea ('toddler diarrhoea')
- irritable bowel syndrome.

Less common causes with growth faltering include:

- parasitosis (*Giardia lamblia, Cryptosporidium*, etc.)
- coeliac disease
- post-enteritis syndrome (small-bowel enteropathy).

'Toddler diarrhoea' (non-specific diarrhoea of childhood)

The exact cause of this diarrhoea is not known, but it may result from an inability of the colon to handle the fluid load. Typically, the patient is a fit and thriving 11- to 24-month-old whose only problem is the presence of watery and runny stools. The stools often contain undigested vegetable material, such as peas and carrots. By definition, if no dietary restrictions are imposed in an attempt to control the diarrhoea, the child continues to gain weight normally. Unfortunately, parents or physicians often discontinue milk, dairy products and other foods; so, eventually, the child may experience faltering growth or actual weight loss. In many cases, an excessive intake of fluids (milk, water, fruit juices and high-carbohydrate drinks) and/or fruit can be identified as a possible cause. Other dietary factors that may contribute include low-fat milk and a low-fat, often very-high-fibre, diet. There is little evidence to suggest that toddler diarrhoea is caused by food sensitivity.

Management
Management centres on reassuring parents that toddler diarrhoea is a transitory condition and will resolve in time. If dietary transgressions are identified, correction to a normal healthy balanced diet with adequate fat intake can improve or resolve the problem completely. In some cases, fibre supplementation may help by giving bulk to the stools.

Gastro-oesophageal reflux

Posseting is a very common phenomenon in babies, especially in the early days/ weeks of life, and would seem more evident in the immature baby. A small amount of milk is frequently brought up when the mother 'winds' the baby. In fact, this very Victorian back-rubbing exercise is often responsible for encouraging milk to leave the stomach and reflux up the oesophagus – clearly, food should never travel in that reverse direction. Incidentally, if a mother simply cuddles her baby against her shoulder, then any 'wind', which seems to preoccupy British and American mothers, will either make an exit when the baby burps or else leave the anus as flatus. Perhaps less aggressive attempts to 'wind' might lower the incidence of reflux!

Reflux, regurgitation and vomiting are not synonyms: reflux and regurgitation are involuntary, in contrast to rumination or vomiting, which involve an active effort.

Postprandial regurgitation, a mild form of gastro-oesophageal reflux (GoR), is a very common paediatric problem that in most instances runs a harmless and self-limited course. Although it effects up to 50% of all babies at two months of age and is still quite frequent at three months, it usually has resolved by six to 12 months. As the infant matures, so do the mechanisms for preventing reflux: for example, the sub-diaphragmatic section of the oesophagus containing the distal sphincter lengthens (Fig. 7.2).

GoR is common in many severely handicapped babies. It can occur in the absence of vomiting – head and upper-trunk arching or hyperextension are useful diagnostic clues.

Excessive regurgitation can result in gastro-oesophageal reflux disease (GoRD) (*see* Boxes 7.1 and 7.2). GoRD can cause apnoea, bradycardia or worsen broncho-pulmonary dysplasia. This disorder is more common in low birthweight babies and among children with cow's-milk allergy, respiratory disease and some disorders of the central nervous system. Owing to regurgitation, poor intake and even feeding refusal, GoRD may result in growth faltering.

With reflux, the feed might need to be thickened with a special starch preparation – e.g. Instant Carobel (Cow & Gate), Vitaquick (Vitaflow), Thick and Easy (Fresenius Kabi) – and the infant positioned in a more upright position after feeds.

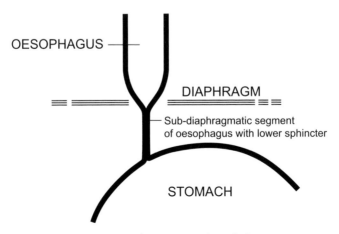

Figure 7.2   Anatomical representation of gastro-oesophageal closure.

Box 7.1   Complications of gastro-oesophageal reflux.

- Oesophagitis
- Oesophageal stricture
- Feeding refusal
- Growth faltering
- Iron-deficiency anaemia
- Haematemesis
- Apnoea
- Dysphonia.

Box 7.2   Symptoms of oesophagitis.

- Irritability
- Feeding refusal
- Interruption of feeding
- Awaking with intense crying
- Haematemesis
- Pounding of the heart (toddlers)
- Abdominal pain
- Chest pain (central or lateral).

Even with breastfeeding such an option can be offered. An H_2 antagonist (e.g. ranitidine) or proton-pump inhibitor (e.g. omeprazole) might be needed. If the condition fails to respond to adequate and prolonged medical therapy, an operation (fundoplication) may be required, although this is rare.

Case study

Jerome was born at 37 weeks' gestation. Within 24 hours of being fed formula, he started to vomit and scream. He would arch his back and appear distressed. The family practitioner offered to refer the baby to a paediatrician, but this was refused by the parents because they were loath for Jerome to undergo a pH oesophageal study, which is an invasive test. They preferred an empirical approach. Thus, the mother was given Thick and Easy, which was added to all of Jerome's formula, and the H_2-receptor antagonist ranitidine was administered twice daily. A marked improvement was observed, and within weeks the thickener was withdrawn. By eight months of age, Jerome was off treatment and symptom-free. Had he not responded to the medication and dietary regimen, further investigations such as a 24-hour pH study and possibly endoscopy with an oesophageal biopsy might have been indicated. Another alternative would have been to offer a thickened formula such as Enfamil AR or SMA Staydown instead of the Thick and Easy.

Milk-sensitive (food-sensitive) colitis

It is certainly possible, yet uncommon, for a newborn to develop, even in the early days of life, inflammation of the large bowel (milk-sensitive colitis). So-called food-sensitive colitis (FSC) is seen much more frequently by paediatricians than is classic ulcerative colitis. FSC is manifested by the presence of small quantities of fresh blood and mucus in the stool. Examination of the inside of the anus/rectum by a very simple bedside technique, which can be carried out by a doctor in a matter of minutes, will confirm the suspicion of bowel inflammation. This phenomenon has even been noted in those solely breastfed: when the mother abstains from milk or dairy products and spices, the problem invariably resolves.

Case study

Daniel, a newborn in a very atopic family, had been successfully breastfed for two months and then switched to standard formula. Within two weeks, eczema developed and his mother noted bright red blood in his mucusy stools. His family doctor very appropriately referred him promptly to a paediatrician. Proctoscopy demonstrated a hyperaemic mucosa and rectal biopsy revealed many eosinophils. These findings confirmed the strong clinical suspicion of milk-induced colitis. Daniel was switched to a hydrolysed milk. Within a few days, the blood disappeared from the stools. In addition, within four weeks, the eczema went into remission. A state registered dietitian played a key role in ensuring the weaning foods were free of milk proteins or their derivatives.

Abdominal pain

It was shown many years ago by a distinguished UK paediatrician, the late John Apley, that as many as one in ten to twelve school-aged children suffer from recurrent abdominal pain (RAP). Dr Apley, in a Bristol-based epidemiological study of 1000 schoolchildren, concluded that the commonest cause was that of emotional stress.

In all, there are said to be more than 80 reasons for a child to have recurrent tummy ache over a period of months if not years, and with at least three episodes a year. There is nothing magical about the value of three, but a definition is needed if we are to use common criteria when discussing patients. The pain is usually in the centre of the abdomen and around the navel. Although there are many explanations for this pain, in our experience – and, indeed, in that of many others – the main causes are:

- constipation
- 'abdominal migraine' or 'migraine equivalent' syndrome
- psychological causes
- lactose intolerance (especially in Asian/Afro-Caribbeans)
- irritable bowel syndrome.

Rarely, it can be caused by a combination of these factors.

Abdominal migraine

It seems odd to use the term 'migraine' — which is derived from the Greek words *hemi* (half) and *kranion* (skull) — when we are focusing upon the abdomen and not the brain, as in classic migraine.

Abdominal migraine is characterised by:

- family history of atopy (in many)
- travel sickness (common)
- pain in the middle of the abdomen
- nausea, if not vomiting
- headache (sometimes)
- blurred vision or flashing lights (rare).

Table 7.1 Tyramine content of cheeses. From Bentley D, Lifschitz C and Lawson M (2002) *Pediatric Gastroenterology and Clinical Nutrition*. Remedica Publishing, London.

Cheese type	Quantity of tyramine ($\mu g/g$)
Cottage cheese	Not detectable
Quark (skimmed-milk soft cheese)	Not detectable
Cream cheese	Not detectable
Curd cheese	Not detectable
Edam	216
Brie	240
Wensleydale	312
Leicester	312
Lancashire	360
Melbury	456
Processed Cheddar	552
Goat cheese	576
Vegetarian Cheddar	601
Derby	648
Mild Cheddar	768
Lymeswold	787
Swiss Emmental	864
Low-calorie Cheddar	912
Mature Cheddar	1036
Italian gorgonzola	1248
Fully matured Cheddar	1440
Danish blue	3840
Blue stilton	4200

By kind permission of S Gray and CS Evans, London.

We believe this condition is caused by the following:

- citrus fruits or juices (especially oranges)
- solid cheeses (not cottage cheese or some of the cream cheeses e.g. Philadelphia)
- chocolate and its derivatives
- caffeine-containing drinks (e.g. tea, coffee, cocoa and cola drinks)
- onions.

In many, there is both a personal and family history of travel sickness and invariably also cephalgic migraine. Tyramine, which is present in many cheeses (*see* Table 7.1), is believed by some to cause the pain.

It is very satisfying for doctors to treat this condition by conservative measures since, in the majority of cases, it so readily responds to the removal of the offending foods or liquids. Parents must remember that the citrus family includes pineapple, lemons, grapefruit, limes and a number of new cultivated hybrid fruits (e.g. tangerines, satsumas, clementines). For adolescents, decaffeinated coffee and tea can be offered as alternative beverages. Carob-containing chocolate substitutes are enjoyed by some. By the age of 13 years, the syndrome disappears.

Lactose intolerance

In many communities, particularly in Asia, Africa, the Caribbean and South America, the milk sugar lactose cannot be tolerated. In fact, there are more people in the world who cannot absorb this carbohydrate than there are those who can. It is said that if any Anglo-Saxon adults are given too large a volume of milk, then many will find that they, in common with non-Caucasians from Africa, will get symptoms.

Intolerance to lactose results from an insufficiency of the lactose-digesting enzyme, lactase. If this enzyme is not present, the disaccharide lactose cannot be hydrolysed into simpler monosaccharides (glucose and galactose). In addition to the inherited disorder, the condition can occur if the small-bowel villi are damaged, as in dietary protein intolerance, or if there is a parasite in the small bowel (e.g. *Giardia lamblia*), or as a consequence of malnutrition.

Secondary lactose intolerance is a transient problem, lasting from a few weeks to six months. Likely symptoms include:

- diarrhoea
- recurrent abdominal pain
- excess flatus
- distension of the abdomen.

When this disorder is suspected, diagnosis can be confirmed by detection of reducing substances in the stool and/or by the hydrogen breath test following a lactose load.

A reduction in the lactose content of the diet may be sufficient to alleviate the pain and other features (*see* Table 7.2).

Table 7.2   Lactose content of foods. From Bentley D, Lifschitz C and Lawson M (2002) *Pediatric Gastroenterology and Clinical Nutrition*. Remedica Publishing, London.

Foods with a high lactose content (>1 g/100 g)	*Foods with a low lactose content (<1 g/100 g)*	*Foods free of lactose*
Milks of all species	Hard cheese	Most coffee
Milk-based desserts	Double/heavy cream	whiteners/creamers
Single/light cream	Butter	Soy milks
Yogurt	Margarines	Margarines prepared
Ice cream	Some processed meat	from vegetable
Some processed infant	and fish dishes	products
savoury dishes	(e.g. burgers, sausages,	Ghee
Creamed soups	fish fingers/sticks,	Oils
Some artificial sweeteners	chicken nuggets)	Cooking fats
Milk chocolate	Toffee	Saccharin
Processed milk/	Filled chocolate products	Cyclamate
cheese-based fruit,	Some fizzy drinks/sodas	Glucose
vegetable and pasta	and 'pop'	Fructose
dishes	Some adult breakfast cereals	Sucrose
White sauce	Some breads	Jam
(sweet and savoury)	Cookies/biscuits/crackers	Jelly
Most infant breakfast	and baked goods	Clear fruit-type
cereals and rusks	Cakes and pastry	sweets and gums
	Pancakes	Gelatin
	Muffins	Most fruit drinks
	Some flavoured	Vegetables
	potato-crisps and	Potatoes
	savoury snacks	Peas
		Beans
		Lentils
		Nuts
		Fruit
		Rice
		Wheat
		Barley
		Oats
		Maize
		Sago
		Semolina
		Tapioca
		Cornflour
		Cornstarch
		Cornmeal
		Some breads
		Most breakfast
		cereals
		Pasta

Constipation

Constipation describes the consistency of a stool and not the frequency of a motion.

There is little doubt that the British in general are unduly concerned not only with their own bowel habits but also with those of their children.

The high sugar content of human milk facilitates soft and frequent stools; as a result, constipation is very rare in breastfed infants. It is more common in those fed infant milks, but babies' bowel habits do vary greatly and parents may have unrealistic expectations of what constitutes 'normal'. Constipation in babies is usually attributable to an inadequate fluid intake, possibly caused by the use of over-concentrated feeds.

There are many non-dietary reasons for constipation in infants and children:

- Parents keen to witness early 'potty' training may be the perpetrators of such. One highly effective method of achieving non-verbal and negative communication with a mother is for an infant to refuse the 'potty'.
- Sometimes, infants retain faeces because they are afraid of the lavatory, particularly when switching from a 'potty'. They might have fears of falling down the toilet: a simple measure, such as providing a special child's seat, may resolve the problem.
- There are some infants who do not find time to empty their bowels. This may be due to a rushed programme of dressing, breakfasting and a scramble to reach school in the morning; or perhaps because more interesting pursuits and options take precedence. In such cases, parents and child must devise a programme whereby, preferably prior to school, a few 'leisurely' minutes are spent in the lavatory – even if the child takes in a book or toy to alleviate the boredom. Establishment of a routine is of great importance in the re-education of bowel habits. However, parents/carers must be helped not to become too obsessive about the child's stools or to make too many enquiries, as this engenders an unhealthy preoccupation, which is counterproductive (Fig. 7.3).
- Often, schoolchildren avoid the school toilet if there is inadequate privacy or the facilities are unclean and the child is sensitive to the dirty conditions.

If severe, it can cause abdominal pain and, at times, small fissure(s) around the anus, which produces such intense discomfort that the child subsequently has a genuine and somatic reason for 'hanging on'.

If a child deliberately soils their underclothes, or hides the stools and is distressed because of unsuccessful efforts to retain the faeces, then evidently we are into the zone of behavioural problems needing the skills of a child/family psychologist or psychiatrist. Frequently, parents do not appreciate that their offspring's anguish is the result of failed efforts to hold back the stool. Perhaps if the British were less preoccupied with overzealous potty training, infants would feel less obliged to hang onto their stools as an act of defiance.

Constipation that persists for years but which was originally noted in the early days of life is regarded much more seriously by doctors. In some circumstances it is due to the absence of nerve ganglion in the bowel lining (Hirschsprung's disease), but this disorder is uncommon. Hypothyroidism and hypercalcaemia can be associated with constipation. Rarely, the malabsorption disorder due to coeliac disease (gluten enteropathy) is characterised not by steatorrhoea but by constipation.

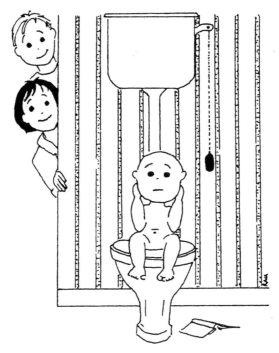

Figure 7.3 Constipation.

To treat constipation, carers should give extra fluid, and/or diluted pure fruit juice if weaning has started. Moreover, those on a weaning diet should have whole-grain cereals such as Weetabix, and puréed fruit and vegetables (for high-fibre-containing foods, *see* Table 4.3). If prune juice added to an infant's diet is ineffective, then, in those aged two years and above, a small daily dose of a laxative such as Senokot (half a teaspoon, 2.5 ml, at night) for a few days should resolve the problem. Short-term use of laxatives will cause no harm, but long-term treatment is not desirable. Docusate, 2.5 mg/kg three times daily, in those of over six months to 12 years is an effective stool-softening agent. To treat anal fissures, apply 2% xylocaine gel to the anus (internally) when the baby or infant is straining and attempting to defecate.

In addition, parents should ensure that their child can sit comfortably on the lavatory seat with both feet on the floor or a platform, in order physically to facilitate defecation. Opening of the bowels depends very much upon being able to strain effectively rather than relying on spontaneous contractions of the intestine. The Valsalva manoeuvre is very important in this respect but is a fact often overlooked by family physicians and paediatricians alike. Imagine trying to pass a stool with both feet dangling above the lavatory floor.

CHAPTER 8

Non-enteric disorders

The crying baby

One of the most important topics a mother will wish to discuss with her family practitioner or baby clinic doctor will relate to the subject of crying. It is not surprising to note that there are numerous reasons why a baby should cry. Clearly, pain, hunger, thirst, tiredness, discomfort, being ill (e.g. earache, fever, etc.) will all cause distress. A breastfed baby can be consoled by being put to the mother's breast even if feeding has just been completed. Mothers need to be reminded that their breasts can soothe and comfort, and not just nourish, their newborn. This puts the baby who is suckled into a more fortunate position than infants on a bottle, who will become obese if fed each time they cry or are distressed.

It is essential to remember that in many respects the baby is a mirror image of the mother. Should the mother be distressed, anxious or weary, then we ought not to be surprised to note a change in the baby's personality. Babies are more sensitive and perceptive to emotional influences in their environment than we give them credit for. An isolated and uncared for young mother, perhaps living in a lonely room, has much to contend with. If she has been abandoned by her partner and family, and perhaps herself was ambivalent about having a baby, we should not be surprised to observe more crying in such a suboptimal situation; indeed, the scene is tragically being set for child abuse. An empathic and able health visitor has a crucial role to play in preventing a crisis situation. Breastfeeding, if mother is not hostile to the concept, will do much to avoid alienation between mother and baby.

A mother who tragically is grieving for the death of someone close, especially if the event was unexpected, would not be predicted to have a bouncy, jovial baby – not in most circumstances. Such emotional confusion is very likely to result in failed lactation. The 'muddled' feelings of joy for the newborn and sadness for the deceased will confuse the baby as well as the mother, and so a crying baby is a predictable outcome. It is not possible to rejoice with the birth of a newborn when recalling memories of a previous miscarriage, or a neonatal or other death.

We have often noticed how a baby's crying pattern after a feed from the breasts can be attributed to the mother's own dairy milk ingestion, and presumed adverse reaction in the infant. If this is the explanation, it will promptly be proven when mother alters her diet by removing the offending food or drink. However, care must be taken to ensure that the mother is not following an unnecessarily restricted diet and is having the appropriate calcium supplement etc. It is also not unusual to see mothers continuing unnecessarily with very restricted diets when no benefit has been seen in the infant. Such dietary restraints are to be avoided unless really justified.

'Cot death' (sudden infant death syndrome)

This is the principal cause of death in those aged between four weeks and 12 months in Western Europe and North America. In the UK, an educational campaign to reduce cot deaths (*see* below), introduced in 1991, has been associated with a 70% decrease in such; nevertheless, more than 300 babies still die annually (Table 8.1). It is important to note that, historically, some deaths labelled as sudden infant death syndrome (SIDS) might have been the result of disease (or child abuse) which the general adult pathologist, in contrast to the paediatric expert, could not detect, and thus the label 'SIDS' with all its implications was given inappropriately. Fortunately, in the UK (as a result of recommendations by The Royal College of Pathologists) and in other developed nations, professional encouragement is now given to ensure that those who die in infancy have a detailed post mortem performed by a paediatric pathologist trained to interpret findings, which might well be subtle. In coming years, this will mean that those so labelled are indeed genuine cases of SIDS.

One possible cause of SIDS is reflux of milk into the oesophagus. Many babies experience reflux. It is thought that the presence of cow's milk in the upper oesophagus – caused by reflux – can stimulate laryngeal receptors and shock the baby, potentially causing SIDS. There is the subjective, but unproven, impression that breastfed babies are at less risk from this tragic condition (Mavis Gunther, 1977). It has also been suggested that a small number of near-miss cot deaths (also known as acute life-threatening events) have been provoked by the presence of cow's milk in the upper oesophagus. We do not claim reflux is a major explanation for SIDS, but this mechanism might be the answer in a number of cases and may constitute yet one more reason for endeavouring to keep babies off cow's-milk formula for as long as possible.

It is quite feasible that in the final analysis there will be more than one finite explanation for the cause of SIDS. It is known that the SIDS rate is highest where the mother is aged under 20 years at the time of the child's birth; also, 60% of all SIDS cases are seen in boys. Formerly, most deaths occurred in winter, but this peak has almost disappeared (2003). Despite earlier teaching, it seems that the safest position for newborns is to sleep on their backs and for them not to be overheated in their cot or bed. A duvet might be potentially dangerous if of a high tog value. Presumably, separate lightweight coverings can be kicked off in older, more mobile infants, and thus lower the body temperature. Sleeping bags for infants are now increasingly popular: they bear set tog values and often are supplied with room thermometers and guidance on how to dress the infant at different temperatures.

Table 8.1 Annual cot deaths in the UK.

Year	Number	Rate per 1000 live births
1997	506	0.67
1998	414	0.55
1999	432	0.59
2000	378	0.54
2001	371	0.53

It is frequently surprising to the parent how little the infant needs to wear. A temperature of 18°C (64°F) is now thought to be the safest and optimal one for the baby's bedroom. Not only is the risk of cot death increased when an infant is overwrapped or overheated, especially if feverish or unwell, but there is a strong relationship between smoking (both before and after birth) and SIDS.

The 'Reduce The Risk' campaign advises nine key steps:

1   A baby should be placed on his/her back to sleep.
2   Smoking in pregnancy (including the father's) should be reduced.
3   Smoking should be forbidden in the baby's room or vicinity.
4   Do not allow the baby to be too hot.
5   The baby's head should be uncovered when asleep.
6   If the baby is unwell, carers must seek medical advice promptly.
7   Parents should not share a bed with the baby if they are smokers, have been drinking, or have been taking drugs or medication that might cause drowsiness or excess tiredness.
8   The cot should be kept in the parental bedroom for the first six months.
9   Parent(s) should avoid falling asleep on a sofa with their baby, or sharing a bed/couch within the first eight weeks of life.

Where a twin has died, the surviving baby must be immediately admitted to hospital for prompt investigation and monitoring, to avoid a second tragedy, although cot deaths have happened within maternity units.

Food intolerance (food allergy)

Is there any topic within paediatrics about which so much nonsense is aired as that relating to food allergy? Quite readily, milk, juices, eggs, wheat and additives of every description are erroneously blamed for a multiplicity of features. Parents need to be made aware that modern food technology is a sophisticated and commercially based industry and that the term 'additives' encompasses a huge spectrum, which includes:

* flavourings – more than 3000 flavourings are used in the British food business
* colouring agents – added to make food visually more attractive, e.g. peas are made greener than their natural colour, which is lessened when processed
* acidulants – said to provide a 'refreshing' quality
* acidity regulators – maintain the acidity
* bulk sweeteners (e.g. glucose, mannitol, sorbitol, xylitol)
* antioxidants
* stabilisers and emulsifiers – avoid separation (food or liquid)
* vitamins
* preservatives – give the food a 'shelf life'
* miscellaneous – includes such products as artificial sweeteners (saccharin, ace-sulfame, aspartame).

So-called experts, including many who lack acceptable professional qualifications, will broadcast to mammoth audiences or answer questions directed to the 'agony aunts' of popular women's magazines and distort or misrepresent the little that is known.

There is no doubt that formerly, doctors, health visitors, midwives and other health carers too rarely invoked foods as the cause of a baby's or infant's problems. However, it would be sad if these days we were to find ourselves attributing too much to allergy. It is only in recent years that academics, in the field of immunology, have seriously acknowledged the role of foods in the causation of several diseases, such as eczema, asthma, some types of inflammation of the bowel, nose and middle ear disease, migraine and, perhaps, behavioural problems. Certainly, with the development of sophisticated blood tests and other techniques, we do find more definite evidence of food allergy. Our concern, if not anxiety, is that it is quite easy to invoke foods as the cause of allergic phenomena (a better term would be 'adverse reactions') without any supporting evidence. However, an observant mother's comments are invaluable in attempting to identify particular suspect foods.

What is food intolerance?

Many people use the term 'allergy' in a very vague sense. For example, if a person eats eggs, fish or perhaps strawberries, and consequently develops swelling and other abnormal and unpleasant features, then this would be interpreted as an 'allergic reaction'. There is no global agreement about this, but most UK allergists would use the label of 'allergy' only if there was an immunoglobulin E (IgE)

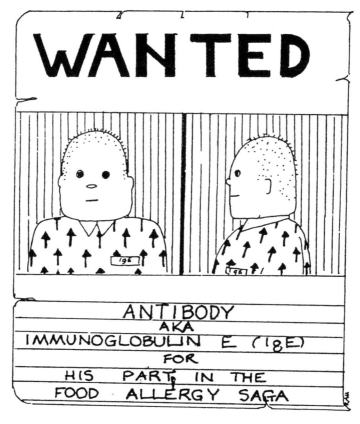

Figure 8.1 Immunoglobulin E – the main culprit in the food allergy saga.

type of activity. IgE is one of several classes of antibody produced by the human body within the immune system and is the main culprit in the food allergy saga (Fig. 8.1). Other classes of antibodies (immunoglobulins) comprise IgA, IgD, IgG and IgM. Antibodies are proteins formed when 'antigens' enter the circulation. An antigen is a substance – usually a protein – that is capable, under appropriate circumstances, of provoking a specific immune response. Antigens may be soluble substances, such as toxins and foreign proteins, or particulate, such as bacteria, viruses and tissue cells.

IgE relates to Type I hypersensitivity reactions, which are mediated by the reaginic or IgE antibody (Fig. 8.2). The antigen forms a complex with the antibody to which it is coupled on the surface of the specialised mast and basophil cells. Then the mechanism is activated and the cells release many complex chemical compounds (e.g. histamine) from within their structures into the bloodstream throughout the body and at localised sites. These substances are responsible for the clinical manifestations that arise, e.g. urticaria ('hives'), asthma and hayfever.

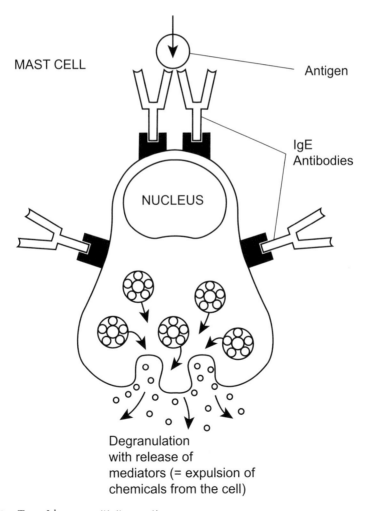

Figure 8.2 Type I hypersensitivity reaction.

Most people form very little IgE but 'atopic' children or adults produce high levels when exposed to an antigen. A food antigen, such as milk protein, does not normally invoke an adverse response, but in those who are vulnerable, the protein behaves as an 'allergen', in that symptoms are caused.

At times it can be difficult to unravel the problem, and, indeed, to be satisfied that there is a genuine disorder and that food is the culprit. Mothers will readily, and understandably, turn their thoughts, perhaps accusatively, towards nutrients as the source of their offspring's ailments. Chemicals may be present not because of a food manufacturer's processing techniques, but simply because they are natural ingredients; for example, oxalic acid in rhubarb, salicylates in vegetables, cyanogens in tapioca, and lectins in beans. The list is endless. Therefore, it is somewhat fatuous to indict the food industry on the premise that babies and children are nutritionally healthier if they avoid 'adulterated' food.

Because of a greater awareness by paediatricians of the whole concept of milk and food intolerance in early life, more cases that formerly were overlooked, yet resolved with the passage of time, are now identified. In our experience, using a very simple inspection test of the inside of the anus (and, at times, taking a tiny pin-headed sample of the rectum for biopsy analysis), cow's milk – even that consumed by a breastfeeding mother – can be identified as being responsible for the development of inflammation in the large bowel (colitis). When, for whatever reason, a decline in breastfeeding arises in various societies, exacerbation of allergic phenomena will be apparent. In some studies, as many as 12% of children have been identified as having adverse reactions, just in the small bowel alone, to milk or dairy products.

Professor Gerrard from Saskatchewan, an international authority on allergy, analysed a group of 81 babies said to be sensitive to foods eaten by the mother while she was breastfeeding, and observed the following symptoms:

- colic ($n = 32$)
- nasal problems ($n = 19$)
- vomiting ($n = 17$)
- diarrhoea ($n = 17$)
- eczema ($n = 13$).

Often, the infant who is sensitive will have some difficulty or perhaps problems in the early weeks. Our anxiety, and this must be stressed, is that mothers will manipulate the baby's diet without expert help. Newborns and young infants are totally dependent upon milk – especially before weaning and, to a lesser extent, during the weaning period – for an adequate intake of nutrients. Therefore, mothers must not carry out elimination diets and exclude essential sources of nutrition and energy unless a qualified person – i.e. a state registered dietitian (SRD) as opposed to one self-appointed (anyone can describe themselves as a nutritionist) – is closely involved in the management.

Why does food intolerance occur?

There is evidence to show genetic factors are involved in the causation of food allergies (Fig. 8.3). If a child has eczema, one or both parents, siblings and/or other relatives on either or both sides of the family invariably have a positive history.

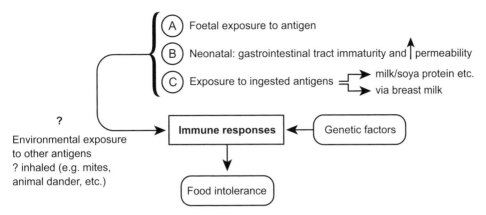

Figure 8.3   Possible pathways of food intolerance. (From Bentley D, Lifschitz C and Lawson M (2002) *Pediatric Gastroenterology and Clinical Nutrition.* Remedica Publishing, London.)

Maybe it is better for both families to have such a track record, to avoid one parent silently if not overtly accusing the other of responsibility in causing the child's disease. Such common recrimination is saddening yet understandable.

Certain immunological factors may predispose a baby to allergy. We know that the small bowel can play an important part in the development of allergic disease. There is some evidence in human newborns of a phenomenon known as 'closure', in which the lining of the small bowel becomes mature and does not absorb proteins or toxins. Until this radical change arises, the infant is at risk of allergen sensitisation. If the baby is premature, the gut lining is less able than that in the term baby to prevent the absorption of cow's-milk proteins, even those derived from the mother's own milk. Furthermore, if the gut lining is damaged because of enteritis resulting from an infection, there is the likelihood of an increased uptake of large molecules. The integrity of the bowel-wall lining is maintained by complex mechanisms. The gut immune system might be inefficient for many reasons, or even lack a particular type of key antibody (secretory IgA) that is normally present. There is animal research evidence to show that prior to birth, when *in utero*, sensitisation to a foreign protein, such as animal milk, can become manifest. If the load of milk proteins (from the cow) is excessive, then this, too, will facilitate adverse reactions. A prudent preventive measure in the optimal management of newborns might be the avoidance of all unmodified cow's-milk proteins until gut immunity systems have reached their peak activity.

Some environmental factors, too, may increase susceptible infants' risk of allergy. If a child is exposed to many non-food allergens, e.g. a cat in the home, a dusty environment, or in a setting where there is much pollen from grass or plants, then the load may be such *in toto* that problems do arise. It has been shown in some investigations that if the allergen challenge is reduced by certain measures in the early weeks of life, eczema and other disorders are less likely to appear.

Prevention of allergy

In the atopic family, the message is quite simple: the newborn ought to avoid all milk except that of the mother, or, if the mother is unable to breastfeed, a hypoallergenic hydrolysed formula should be used. Ingestion of other milk, even one teaspoon (5 ml) or less of such, before the baby has a mature bowel immune system, may be enough to sensitise. Breastfeeding should continue for as long as possible and weaning delayed until six months of age. There is disagreement in respect of the time that potentially allergenic foods should be avoided from the infant's diet; however, it would seem prudent to initially avoid cow's milk products, eggs, wheat and soy foods.

Dietary management

Almost every food ever consumed has been cited as an allergen in the medical literature. Foods and additives commonly implicated in adverse reactions are listed in Table 8.2. For products containing milk, see Box 1.2 (p. 22). Food dyes are not allergic per se, but may become so when linked to large protein molecules. Other substances undergo transformation to allergens only after they have been altered by the digestive systems of the body. Cooking or food processing can also affect allergenicity: a hard-boiled egg is less allergenic than a raw one. Certain foods may not give rise to any problems when eaten in isolation but become allergenic when

Table 8.2 Foods/additives potentially provoking adverse reactions.

Disease spectrum	Foods/additives most commonly implicated
Migraine	Chocolate, cheese and dairy products, citrus fruits, alcohol, tea, coffee, pork, fish, shellfish, wheat, vegetables (especially onions), fatty foods
Urticaria and angioedema	Nuts, eggs, fish, shellfish, yeasts, pork, chocolate, banana, berry fruits (particularly strawberries), salicylates, azo dyes, antioxidants, preservatives, flavourings
Upper respiratory tract (nasal congestion and catarrh)	Milk and dairy products
Asthma and eczema	Milk, cheese, dairy products, egg, chocolate, nuts, fish, shellfish, chicken, beef, beans, yeast, azo dyes
Asthma	Tartrazine, benzoic acid, sulphites
Gastrointestinal	Milk, dairy products, egg, fish, shellfish, chicken, wheat, rice, soy, pork
Hyperkinesis	Salicylates, colourings, flavourings, emulsifiers and stabilisers

taken in combination. Allergy to one food is likely to produce cross-reactions with biologically related products. If eggs are not tolerated, chicken should be suspected until proved otherwise; similarly, beef and veal in milk protein allergy, and broad beans, peas and lentils where peanuts are known to be allergenic. The dose is sometimes important — for example, one strawberry might be tolerated, whereas a punnet of such could produce urticaria.

Mother keeping a diary of symptoms and noting the types of drinks and foods consumed can often identify the foodstuff responsible for the allergy. The food scrutiny should cover at least the 48-hour period immediately prior to the appearance of the problem; however, even this may be too short a time to elucidate some of the delayed reactions. Mothers are very ill-advised to go in for dietary manipulation, especially elimination diets, without skilled help. This is because of the complexity of the subject, and the need to supply all of the child's nutrients, which are quite extensive and must include protein, carbohydrate, fat, minerals, trace elements and vitamins.

If the dietitian and doctor cannot identify the suspected culprit food(s), then rarely a 'few foods diet' may be implemented. This must be closely supervised by an SRD, as such very restricted diets require micronutrient supplements and must not exceed six weeks' duration.

Food additives and hyperactivity (hyperkinesis)

Attention-deficit hyperactivity disorder (ADHD) is a behavioural syndrome characterised by restlessness, impulsivity and poor concentration. It affects 1%–2% of children in the UK. It is much more common in boys than in girls. These children have insufficient dopamine in the central nervous system and excess of their dopamine transporter. Most cases are due to genetic factors — probably polygenic in nature.

Paediatricians, dietitians and nutritionists seem to polarise into either ardent supporters or vehement opponents of Dr Feingold's theory, which postulates that hyperkinesis (which is said to affect up to one in 10 of American children) can be managed by eliminating additives from the diet. His theory was based on his experience as an American paediatrician and not on carefully carried out research. Egger, in an oft-cited controlled trial in London, demonstrated that sugar was implicated in causing behavioural problems within a small group of children. Yet, within limits, many of the features of ADHD, alone or even in combination, can appear in normal children. Moreover, the evidence pointing to so-called 'natural salicylates', present in fruits and vegetables, and dyes and colouring agents (e.g. tartrazine and benzoic acid) as being responsible for the alleged disorder is anecdotal. Although in the US much support has emanated from parents and the media for the validity of the Feingold hypothesis, it can be imprudent to too readily lay the blame on salicylates, colouring agents or 'E' numbers.

Our experience over many years has shown that the very families with many stresses to bear and difficulties of a psychosocial nature will too easily attribute much, if not everything, to the child's diet. We all need to keep an open mind, but it is important, if we are not to allow medical science to fall into disrepute, for us to see established data in a particular child that show natural salicylates etc., and not genes combined with family stress and strife, to be the true causative agents.

Notwithstanding the aforementioned, we do believe that some parents and carers have noted a genuine association between abnormal patterns of childhood behaviour and specific nutrients. Many children become 'high' when they drink excessive (or, at times, modest) volumes of drinks containing caffeine, such as Coca Cola (35–46 mg in 360 ml), Pepsi Cola (35–38 mg in 360 ml) and, more notably, cocoa (50 mg in 240 ml). More informative packaging and attempts by food and drink manufacturers to conform to new EU guidelines will enable families to see just what the crisps, fizzy drinks, confectionery, etc., do contain (Fig. 8.4). However, the apparently same product can differ in constituents according to the country of origin. Therefore, parents need to be vigilant where they are convinced 'X' can upset their child, especially when out of their homeland.

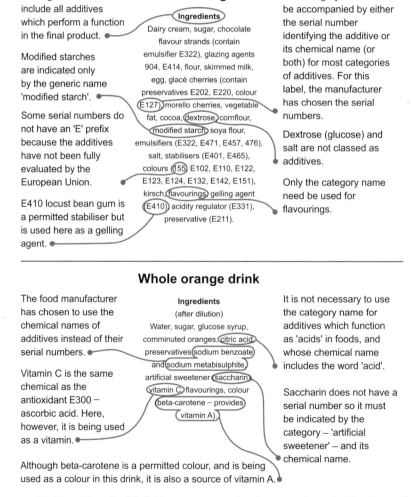

Black Forest gateau

The ingredients list must include all additives which perform a function in the final product.

Modified starches are indicated only by the generic name 'modified starch'.

Some serial numbers do not have an 'E' prefix because the additives have not been fully evaluated by the European Union.

E410 locust bean gum is a permitted stabiliser but is used here as a gelling agent.

Ingredients

Dairy cream, sugar, chocolate flavour strands (contain emulsifier E322), glazing agents 904, E414, flour, skimmed milk, egg, glacé cherries (contain preservatives E202, E220, colour E127) morello cherries, vegetable fat, cocoa, dextrose, cornflour, modified starch, soya flour, emulsifiers (E322, E471, E457, 476), salt, stabilisers (E401, E465), colours (155) E102, E110, E122, E123, E124, E132, E142, E151), kirsch, flavourings, gelling agent (E410) acidity regulator (E331), preservative (E211).

The category name must be accompanied by either the serial number identifying the additive or its chemical name (or both) for most categories of additives. For this label, the manufacturer has chosen the serial numbers.

Dextrose (glucose) and salt are not classed as additives.

Only the category name need be used for flavourings.

Whole orange drink

The food manufacturer has chosen to use the chemical names of additives instead of their serial numbers.

Vitamin C is the same chemical as the antioxidant E300 – ascorbic acid. Here, however, it is being used as a vitamin.

Ingredients
(after dilution)

Water, sugar, glucose syrup, comminuted oranges, citric acid, preservatives sodium benzoate and sodium metabisulphite, artificial sweetener saccharin, vitamin C flavourings, colour beta-carotene – provides vitamin A).

It is not necessary to use the category name for additives which function as 'acids' in foods, and whose chemical name includes the word 'acid'.

Saccharin does not have a serial number so it must be indicated by the category – 'artificial sweetener' – and its chemical name.

Although beta-carotene is a permitted colour, and is being used as a colour in this drink, it is also a source of vitamin A.

Figure 8.4   Understanding the label. Here is an example of an ingredients list. It shows what the manufacturer has used to produce the food, in order of the amount used; the first ingredient listed is used in the greatest amount, the last one in the smallest amount.

Box 8.1 Main additives thought to be responsible for hyperkinesis.

102	Tartrazine
110	Sunset yellow
122	Carmoisine
123	Amaranth
124	Ponceau 4R
127	Erythrosine
210	Benzoic acid
211	Sodium benzoate
320	Butylated hydroxyanisole (BHA)
321	Butylated hydroxytolouene (BHT)

Enthusiasts for the Feingold (Kaizer-Permanente) diet believe numerous additives should be excluded. For a comprehensive list, see the book *E for Additives*. A much better and more objective evaluation, written with greater clarity, is to be found in *Understanding Additives*. Major suspect numbers are listed in Box 8.1.

Compliance with the Feingold hypothesis entails the removal from the diet of natural salicylates. Not surprisingly, food legislation varies globally, and synthetic salicylate is a permitted food additive in the US but is not used in the UK. Foods that may contain natural salicylates or additives are listed in Box 8.2.

Box 8.2 Salicylates and additives in foods.

Foods that contain natural salicylates

Vegetables	Cucumbers, peas, tomatoes
Fruits and nuts	Almonds, apples, apricots, bananas, berry fruits (cherries, grapes, raspberries, strawberries), currants, oranges and similar (citrus) fruits, peaches, prunes, raisins, rhubarb, sultanas

Foods that may contain additives

Protein foods	Canned, dehydrated and frozen meat or fish products; fresh products coated with breadcrumbs, such as ham and fried fish; sausages; luncheon meats; burgers
Cereal products	Breakfast cereals; bought cakes, biscuits, bread, cookies and pastry; cake mixes; popcorn; non-wholemeal pastas and noodles; tinned spaghetti in sauce
Dairy products	Ice cream, milk shakes, processed cheese, dessert mixes and puddings, flavoured yoghurts, magarines

Confectionery	Hard and soft sweets or candies; chocolate containing fruit or almonds; mints; cough sweets; fruit squash drinks; carbonated or 'fizzy' drinks; chewing gum; jams and lemon curd
Miscellaneous	Canned and dehydrated soups; sauces, vinegar, pickles, salad dressings; crisps and similar products; vegetables in sauce (e.g. baked beans); beer, wine and cider
Non-food items	Aspirin and similar drugs; toothpaste, mouthwashes, throat lozenges; perfumes; any pills or tablets with coloured surround; coloured medicines or cough mixtures

Children with ADHD often have co-morbidities, e.g. dyslexia, dyspraxia, part of the autistic spectrum, and antisocial behaviour. Methylphenidate (Ritalin) and dexamphetamine have been used successfully in selected cases. These powerful drugs must be introduced and monitored by expert child psychiatrists with the appropriate expertise. Newer modified-release preparations such as Concerta XL may achieve better control of symptoms. Some experts in neurophysiology claim these children are depleted of omega-3 and to fatty acids. When this deficiency is corrected an improvement is seen in a proportion of cases.

Case study

Saul had been a calm and contented baby until he reached infancy. At three years of age, he developed a strong liking for Coca Cola. His mother became concerned about his aggression with his other, younger sibling, manifest shortly after he had drunk a large glass of this caffeine-containing drink. With age, he became tolerant of small volumes of cola drinks, but could not tolerate chocolate. Nutritional counselling achieved prompt resolution of his restlessness, poor attention span and anger. However, investigators now believe that ADD and ADHD is polygenic and that dietary manipulation will be the answer in only a minority of cases.

Obesity

> Obesity is harmful to the body and makes it sluggish, disturbs its functions and hinders its movements.
>
> The Medical Aphorisms of Moses Maimonides (1135–1204)

Obesity is the most common nutritional problem in the industrialised world. The incidence and severity of obesity have increased yearly in alarming proportions. Paediatricians and dietitians are most concerned about the topic of obesity because there is considerable evidence linking some adult disorders such as heart and cardio-vascular disease with excessive weight in childhood. Moreover, we are now seeing children with type 2 diabetes and even a number needing overnight ventilation with continuous positive airways pressure (CPAP) due to sleep apnoea. Research has shown that 80% of obese nine-year-olds will be obese at 35 years of age.

Obesity in children can also cause many psychological problems. These include bullying, low self-esteem, depression (particularly among girls), problems social-ising, and even poorer educational attainment, lower income and less likelihood of marriage. It is prudent to recall that 30% of obese adolescent girls manifest binge-eating disorders.

Parents can feel entrapped – especially mothers. As the supplier of all nutrition, mothers are readily hurt, if not guilt-ridden, when told their children must lose weight. Clearly, it seems to reflect upon their caring standards. Thus, doctors ought to adopt a gentle, empathic attitude with the mothers who want slimmer infants, but feel obliged to respond to their offspring's increased food demands, which cannot readily be curtailed.

Definition

Overweight and obesity are conditions in which there is too much body fat, and are best defined using the body-mass index (BMI), where $BMI = weight/height^2$. The BMI charts now available for children are essential for all practices. The latest version in paediatrics has two extra lines near the 91st and 99th centiles, which are the new International Obesity Task Force cut-offs for overweight and obesity, respectively. Previously, obesity was defined as a weight of 120% or more of that which is normal for height.

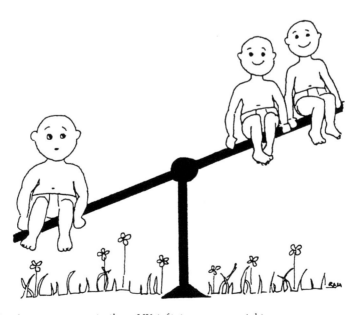

Figure 8.5   As many as one in three UK infants are overweight.

Prevalence

The 1999 Health Survey for England revealed that 44% of men and 33% of women are overweight, with a further 19% of men and 21% of women being classified as clinically obese. In children, the frequency of overweight ranged from 22% at six years of age to 31% at age 15 years, and that of obesity ranged from 10% at six years to 17% at age 15. One study showed that up to one in three English infants were overweight (Fig. 8.5). A report published in *The Lancet* in 2002 stated that the rates of obesity in children have increased 2.0–2.8 fold over 10 years. Social class is inversely related to the prevalence of obesity. A study performed in a deprived area of London found that 35% of adolescents were overweight, with 20% being obese: this was across all ethnic groups.

Aetiology

Both conditions arise because the energy intake is greater than the expenditure (i.e. there is a positive energy balance). Genetic, environmental and psychological factors are all thought to play a role in the aetiology of such.

Obesity is more common in those children who have fat parents. If one parent is overweight, there is a fourfold probability of the child having a similar problem, but this increases to eight- to 10-fold if both parents are obese. Genetic factors are thought to determine relative vulnerability to weight gain, which is then influenced by environmental factors. One investigator has found that overweight dogs are more likely to have obese, rather than slim, owners, which suggests that people differ in the level of obesity they find acceptable both in their families and for their pets.

The most recent discoveries regarding obesity are related to the hormone leptin and the identification of certain genes in animal models. Leptin, which is mainly expressed in adipocytes, contributes to the regulation of body weight. Only a few obese humans have been identified with mutations in the leptin or leptin receptor genes; however, most cases of obesity in humans are associated with high leptin levels. Thus, in humans, obesity may represent a state of leptin resistance.

Eating habits and lifestyle play an important part in the development of obesity. Causal factors include:

- parents being poor role models with respect to the type and amount of food bought and consumed
- an excessive intake of foods with a high fat and/or sugar content
- preference for snacking
- reduced physical activity.

Children regularly snack on energy-dense foods and eat little fruit and vegetables. They may spend their spare time playing computer games or watching television, and only half walk or cycle to school. The National Diet and Nutrition Survey (published in 2000) found that 40% of boys and 60% of girls studied failed to meet health education authority recommendations that young people should participate in physical activity of at least moderate intensity for one hour daily. In addition it was observed that children's consumption of fruit and vegetables had been falling for the past 20 years and that half of those surveyed had eaten neither fruit nor vegetables in a given week.

Contrary to earlier theories, not all obese children eat excessively. Overweight children are less active than their leaner counterparts, and this pattern of reduced physical activity is thought to be an important factor. Among adults, the average recorded energy intake in the UK has declined substantially as obesity rates have escalated, which suggests that sedentary lifestyles are a significant issue.

One investigator reported that the most important factor associated with obesity in two-year-olds was their birth weight. In addition, there is some evidence that breastfeeding seems to offer protection against the development of obesity. This piece of data needs to be put to overweight mothers in the antenatal period if they are opposed to the prospect of using their own milk. Although the majority of obese babies (more than 80%) lose their excess fat beyond infancy, fat babies have a greater likelihood than their thinner peers of having this problem in childhood or adolescence. Therefore, those in the healthcare professions must do all they can to ensure mothers are aware of the potential hazards of obesity if present in the first year of life.

In one study, 60% of bottle-fed infants put on too much weight in the first year compared with only 19% of breastfeeders. Although obesity is caused by many factors, we need to ask why a given mother has offered her infant more milk than is needed. Every cry might be interpreted as a plea for another feed. Very often, food, in both adults and children, is used for comfort, particularly at times of stress.

Prevention

Prevention of obesity is achievable and is evidently preferable to treatment. Children are at increased risk of obesity if they come from families where:

- one or both parents are overweight
- siblings are overweight
- the diet is known to be unsuitable
- much time is spent doing sedentary activities
- income is low.

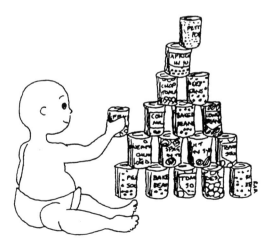

Figure 8.6   Extra play might compensate for a baby being deprived of excessive feeds.

Extra play might compensate for a baby being deprived of excessive feeds (Fig. 8.6); high-calorie snacks should be avoided and the diet should contain plenty of fruit and vegetables.

Management

The core principles for management are as follows:

- Energy intake should be reduced and healthy eating encouraged (*see* Table 8.3).
- Sedentary behaviour should be decreased to less than two hours per day – this includes watching television and computer activity.
- Physical activity should be increased to 30–60 minutes a day.
- For children of primary school age or below, the main responsibility rests with the parents – they should provide healthy food choices and thus help their children to avoid high-energy foods.
- Lifestyle change involves making small gradual changes. (Behaviour modification programmes).
- Family-based protocols are necessary for treatment to succeed.

Table 8.3 Dietary recommendations for the management of overweight or obesity. To reduce energy intake and encourage healthy eating, choose meals from the foods listed in the first column* and avoid those listed in the second.

Choose	*Limit*
Lean meat	Sucrose
Poultry	Sorbitol
Fish	Glucose
Eggs	Jam
Vegetables – all varieties of green and root vegetables and salads	Marmalade
	Honey
Fruit – all varieties of fresh fruit or fruit canned in natural juice	Treacle
	Syrup
Wholegrain cereals – rice, pasta, chappati and breads	Sweets
	Fruit squash, cordials, fizzy drinks
Drinks – low-calorie squash, cordial and fizzy drinks; unsweetened fruit juice (limited to one glass/day); tea and coffee without sugar; unthickened soups.	Chocolate
	Sweet biscuits
	Cream
	Fried foods
	Crisps
	Cakes, pastries
	Pies
	Proprietary slimming and diabetic foods except sugar-free low-energy drinks

*The ideal plate should have two-fifths of it covered by vegetables, two-fifths by starchy foods and one-fifth by protein foods. Five portions of fruit and vegetables should be taken per day (minimum).

Precise treatment will depend upon the age of the child and the severity of the obesity.

In most obese children, weight maintenance is an acceptable goal. Weight loss should be limited to those being cared for by secondary care services (SIGN guidelines, 2003) and then the maximum weight loss recommended is 0.5 kg per month. The SIGN guidelines state the following children should be referred to hospital or community paediatric consultants:

- those with serious obesity-related morbidity that requires weight loss
- children with a suspected underlying medical cause of obesity, including all children under 24 months of age who are severely obese (BMI > 99.6th centile).

Parents, especially mothers, should receive help from a health visitor interested in the topic or a family practitioner. In some areas of the UK and US, and no doubt elsewhere in the West, specialised obesity clinics exist, usually in a non-school setting, and have a moderate success rate. Recent work in both the UK and US, which has been school-based, failed to show that intervention programmes improve BMI (except one study showing girls' BMI improved), although there were changes in eating patterns.

Clinicians must remind mothers that at the time of weaning, milk intake can be controlled at about one pint a day (approximately 500 ml, with a minimum of 300 ml). It can be stressful for parents because although they want a slimmer infant, they become concerned that no increase in weight has taken place perhaps over many weeks or indeed months, as the child's weight is still excessive allowing for the height. However, dietary restrictions can be hazardous, and SRDs must be involved to ensure major nutrients are supplied and no deficiency disorders arise. Mothers must avoid adding sugars to feeds; water or dilute juices can be used after a meal. High-energy foods, such as those rich in fats, can be replaced by those with a lower energy density, e.g. fruits, vegetables, lean meats, fish and wholegrain cereals (*see* Table 8.3). The government has created a '5-a-day' programme aimed at increasing fruit and vegetable consumption. Those aged 4–6 years in English state schools will be entitled to a free piece of fruit each day. One million children now receive this fruit from National Lottery funding (2004).

In our experience, dietary control is futile until the mother is truly convinced that it is necessary, and indeed beneficial, in both the short and long term.

Heart disease

Dietary, genetic and other factors such as birth weight are associated with the high incidence of heart disease that occurs in the Western world. As a consequence of one health visitor's enthusiasm for data-collecting 50 years ago in Hertfordshire, it has recently been shown that in males there is an important correlation between weight at one year of age and subsequent death rates from ischaemic heart disease: the lower the weight at 12 months, the higher the mortality rate in adulthood. A number of other studies have demonstrated that there is a link between small babies and raised blood pressure in adulthood as well as elevated serum cholesterol – particularly low-density lipoprotein (LDL) cholesterol – and abnormal handling of blood glucose (impaired glucose tolerance) in later years. Evidence suggests that it is the poor foetal growth which is related to the blood pressure problem in adulthood.

Professor David Barker, a distinguished epidemiologist, talks of a 'new model for the causation of coronary heart disease'. Previously, the problems of coronary heart disorders were associated with a sedentary lifestyle and smoking, but now the new concept focuses attention upon undernutrition of the fetus within the uterus. Therefore, not only is the smoking mother damaging her own health and jeopardising the immediate wellbeing of her newborn, but in having a growth-retarded baby she is unknowingly laying the seed for major ailments in later decades. The many aspects of the causative components are complex and it is too simplistic for us to believe that reducing the cholesterol intake in a baby or infant will prevent the development in early adult life of heart and blood vessel disease. Furthermore, despite the anxiety related to fears of a high cholesterol intake, the

Table 8.4 Normal serum* cholesterol levels in childhood and adolescence/early adulthood in the UK.

	Mean		5th percentile		95th percentile	
	mmol/l	mg/dl	mmol/l	mg/dl	mmol/l	mg/dl
Males + females†						
$1\frac{1}{2}$–$2\frac{1}{2}$ years	4.39	170	3.01	116	5.72	222
$2\frac{1}{2}$–$3\frac{1}{2}$ years	4.42	171	3.18	123	5.68	2.20
Males						
$3\frac{1}{2}$–$4\frac{1}{2}$ years†	4.36	169	3.23	125	5.46	211
$4\frac{1}{2}$–6 years‡	4.11	160	2.94	114	5.11	198
7–10 years	4.40	170	3.00	116	5.59	216
11–14 years	4.13	160	2.54	98	5.50	213
15–18 years	3.95	153	2.85	110	5.08	196
Females						
$3\frac{1}{2}$–$4\frac{1}{2}$ years†	4.45	172	3.06	118	5.67	219
$4\frac{1}{2}$–6 years‡	4.61	178	2.87	111	6.22	240
7–10 years	4.43	171	2.72	105	6.02	233
11–14 yers	4.26	165	2.99	116	5.49	212
15–18 years	4.20	162	2.90	112	5.44	210

* Serum values = plasma levels × 1.03
† Adapted from Gregory JR, Collins DL, Davies PS *et al* (1995) *National Diet & Nutrition Survey: children aged $1\frac{1}{2}$–$4\frac{1}{2}$ years*. HMSO, London.
‡ Adapted from Gregory JR and Lowe S (2000) *National Diet & Nutrition Survey: young people aged 4 to 18 years*. The Stationery Office, London.

synthesis of cholesterol in the liver is much more important in influencing the blood level than is the amount of dietary cholesterol consumed.

Special complexes of lipids and apolipoproteins – LDLs – are the major transport proteins for cholesterol, and are important in the development of the disease in the arteries, which can date from childhood. A famous study often quoted was carried out in Framingham in America and demonstrated an association between a high level of LDL cholesterol and risk of subsequent heart disease. Large population studies have shown that risk factors for coronary heart disease include low levels of high-density lipoprotein (HDL). The normal serum cholesterol levels in children and adolescents are listed in Table 8.4.

Prevention

There is evidence that reducing LDL cholesterol and increasing HDL cholesterol, by dietary manipulation, is effective in preventing the deposition of fats etc. in the walls of the arteries. Children at particular risk of developing arterial disease, e.g. where there has been the death of a father at a young age (under 50 years) from coronary heart disease and families known to have high levels of cholesterol and/ or triglyceride, must be investigated (Table 8.5).

An improved diet in children and adolescents might be reflected in lower fat levels in the blood in adulthood. Even though cow's milk is a source of animal fats, it should be continued until the age of five years because of its energy density and vitamin A and D content. If an expert in dietetics has recommended skimmed milk before the age of five years, it is essential to ensure that the diet is nutritionally complete. Semi-skimmed milk can be introduced from the age of two years.

A preventive diet would be low in saturated dietary fats (providing under 10% of the total energy content), high in soluble fibre (beans, lentils, pulses and fruits),

Table 8.5   Risk factors for premature heart disease in children. (Adapted from Ose L and Tonstad S (1995) The detection and management of dyslipidaemia in children and adolescents. *Acta Paediatr.* **84**: 1213–15.)

Cholesterol level mmol/l	Sex	Family history of premature heart disease	Risk category
5.3–6.9	M & F	No family history	Low
	F	History of early CHD in men only	Low
	M	History of early CHD	Moderate
	F	History of early CHD	Moderate
7.0–9.9	F	No family history	Low
	M	No family history	Moderate
	M & F	History of early CHD	High
≥10.0	F	No family history	Moderate
	M	No family history	High

CHD = coronary heart disease.

contain at least five portions of fruit and vegetables daily, and include two portions of oily fish per week.

Faltering growth

Faltering growth, or failure to thrive, is estimated to affect as many as 5% of children in the UK. The majority of cases occur before the age of 18 months, when growth is rapid and nutrient requirements are high. The term 'failure to thrive' is now out of fashion as it implies failure of wellbeing in addition to growth failure, which parents might interpret as being judgmental.

Definition

Growth faltering describes growth velocity that is less than that to be expected for a child's age and size. Because it describes velocity, it cannot be diagnosed on the basis of a single measurement in isolation. There is no commonly agreed definition for faltering growth, although a drop of 0.67 SD scores or two to three centile bands on standard growth charts have been suggested. Accurately plotted growth centile charts for weight, height and head circumference are essential tools for diagnosis and monitoring. These can be aided by the use of thrive lines, slow growth monitoring charts and BMI charts. These are all available from the Child Growth Foundation.

Effect of faltering growth

Despite intensive input from healthcare professionals, most children with faltering growth do not entirely achieve their projected weight or height. Some short-term studies have described cognitive defects in young children with faltering growth, but there appear to be no major long-term adverse effects.

Causes

Reasons for inadequate nutrient intake can be separated into the categories below:

A. Clinical conditions
• Increased requirements, e.g. cystic fibrosis
• Increased losses, e.g. gastroenteritis
• Failure to absorb, e.g. cow's or soy milk protein enteropathy
• Failure to utilise, e.g. metabolic disease
• Gut dysmotility.

B. Psychosocial difficulties
• Poverty
• Inadequate parenting skills
• Poor feeding environment
• Behavioural problems
• Early adverse feeding experiences, e.g. nasogastric feeding or gastro-oesophageal reflux (GoR)
• Maternal depression.

C. Feeding difficulties
- Developmental delay
- GoR
- Oral-motor dysfunction
- Communication disorders.

The literature states that about 5% of children with faltering growth will have an organic disorder. However, in our experience and particularly that of a large multidisciplinary feeding clinic, when dealing with chronic and severe failure to thrive, an organic cause is often found. Dysmotility disorders affecting the swallowing and GoR can readily be missed. Despite that, even when the disorder is successfully treated, the child will frequently continue to associate eating with discomfort or pain.

Management

The dietitian will usually increase the energy density of meals. This can simply be done by adding extra oil, cheese, cream, butter and fats to foods. It may include use of a high-calorie formula (up to 18 months) or supplemented drink in those over 12 months of age. In addition, it is essential to ensure that the micronutrient intake is adequate. An age-appropriate multivitamin and mineral supplement may well be indicated and also relieves parental anxiety in respect of the inadequacy of the former diet. Advice might be needed regarding behavioural feeding techniques (*see* Chapter 4).

A multidisciplinary team in persistent cases is invaluable. A home visit might achieve far more than attending a hospital or community clinic. In the absence of such a team, a joint home visit by the health visitor, dietitian, and speech and language therapist can be very useful.

Monitoring

Infants and children with faltering growth should be weighed and measured at regular intervals to ensure they have not regressed.

Recovery is identified when the child's weight returns to within one centile band of the original growth trajectory.

Iron-deficiency anaemia

Iron-deficiency anaemia is the commonest form of malnutrition globally, affecting 43% of the world's children. In the UK, the National Diet and Nutrition Survey of 1995 identified that 12% of a nationally representative sample of children aged 18–30 months had a haemoglobin value of less than 110 g/l. Other UK studies suggest a prevalence of 5%–40%, and it is more common in the underprivileged and ethnic minority communities.

Aetiology

The development of iron-deficiency anaemia in babies and infants will be influenced by the presence of this condition in the mother during pregnancy, the maturity of the newborn, and dietary factors. It is important that iron-deficient pregnant women receive iron treatment (as well as folic acid pre-conceptually) to ensure there is a transfer of this essential metal to the fetus.

The main cause of iron deficiency in the first six months of life is prematurity, leading to inadequate accumulation in the newborn's iron stores. Low birthweight (LBW) babies are also at risk. Premature babies should be iron supplemented if breastfed. The specialised LBW milks for preterm infants – e.g. Prematil (Milupa), SMA Low Birthweight (Wyeth) and Osterprem (Farleys) – all are fortified with iron.

The term infant has a store of iron that will last until about six months of age. After this time, those who are exclusively breastfed – and, even more so, those who erroneously are given whole cow's milk (doorstep milk) – will receive insufficient iron to maintain adequate stores. The iron in breast milk is well absorbed, but the concentration is only modest. Breastfeeding without complementing with iron-rich foods becomes an increasing risk factor for iron deficiency in the second six months of life. Cow's milk not only has a low concentration of iron, but the iron is poorly absorbed and additional sources must be obtained from weaning foods. All standard baby milk formulas in the UK and US are fortified with iron. The routine demineralised whey-based preparations (i.e. 'highly modified'), such as Premium (Cow & Gate), SMA Gold (Wyeth) and Aptamil (Milupa), as well as the 'modified' milks, such as Plus (Cow & Gate), SMA White (Wyeth) and Milumil (Milupa), all have an iron component. It is important to note that the soy milks produced for infants, such as Formula S (Cow & Gate), Wysoy (Wyeth) and Prosobee (Mead Johnson), too, contain iron.

Enthusiasts of goat's milk (*see* p. 44) need to observe that it has, at source, even less iron than the low amount to be found in cow's milk. Moreover, goat's milk, in common with cow's milk, is low in vitamins A and D. Although it has a low folic acid content, this deficiency as well as the iron is corrected in the UK by the goat milk formula producers.

Some weaning foods are high in iron (e.g. liver, red meat, egg yolk and cereals). However, even though foods such as vegetables or fortified cereals might be rich in iron, it does not mean that this is absorbed as readily as the iron in red meat. In the former, the iron is present in its non-haem form, whereas the latter contains haem iron (*see* Chapter 4). Today, non-haem iron sources account for 96% of total iron intake. The bioavailability of non-haem iron is influenced by dietary factors. Substances such as phytates (found in cereals and bread) and phosphates (present in milk, eggs and some vegetables) can form compounds with non-haem iron, which then inhibits absorption of such. The absorption of non-haem iron in foods is increased if vitamin C is consumed at the same time. Also, the amount of iron absorbed from the child's bowel will be influenced by the presence and severity of the shortage of iron: poor iron status results in greater iron absorption.

Prevention and treatment

In Western children, iron deficiency is almost always the result of dietary factors and thus is preventable. Sound nutritional advice from health visitors, baby clinics and general practitioners is vital in this regard. As discussed previously, dietary factors that increase risk include:

- early use of cow's milk (before 12 months) as a main milk drink
- delayed weaning
- weaning diet containing insufficient iron-rich foods, particularly highly absorbable haem iron sources (meat, chicken and fish)
- poor intake of foods rich in vitamin C
- excessive reliance on milks or other fluids in the second year of life.

Preventive options include:

- introducing iron-rich foods, particularly meat, chicken and fish, early into the weaning diet
- if the parents prefer their child to be vegetarian, emphasise the most absorbable sources of non-haem iron (such as grains) and enhancing the absorption of such by taking in foods rich in vitamin C at the same meal
- avoidance of tea (which contains tannin), as this inhibits non-haem iron absorption
- use of follow-on formula in the second year of life.

As many parents will know, ensuring a toddler eats an adequate and healthy diet can pose a considerable challenge. Many factors can impede good nutrition, including faddiness, food refusal, poor mealtime routine, laziness chewing, small appetite, parental anxiety and preference for drinks rather than food.

The iron in follow-on milks will prevent iron deficiency in those on inadequate weaning diets. In a study of children over one year of age living in an inner-city housing estate in Birmingham, it was demonstrated that those who consumed follow-on formula did not become anaemic whereas 26% of those on cow's milk did.

Parents invariably believe, albeit erroneously, that standard vitamin drops for children contain iron.

In the UK, iron is not recommended routinely for healthy newborns but is commonly prescribed for the premature baby and in other specific medical conditions.

As is the case for many comparable metals, and, indeed, vitamins, exposure of the body to excessive amounts can be quite harmful. So, if iron is prescribed, it should be only when there is laboratory evidence to convince the doctor that anaemia is present. Parents must always be advised that accidental ingestion of iron in infants – an all-too-common occurrence – has been responsible for death when large amounts have been consumed. Iron is only one of many medications that should be dispensed in 'child-proof' containers.

Case study

The diet of Russell, aged two years, was made up of large quantities of doorstep milk, yoghurts, biscuits, bananas and little else. His pallor and fatigue brought him eventually to the attention of the family doctor. A blood test revealed a haemoglobin of only 8 g/100 ml (minimum at this age is 11 g/100 ml) and a blood film showed a hypochromic, microcytic picture. After three months of oral iron, his colour, fervour and general wellbeing were much improved. A repeat test confirmed an improvement. The second test was justified to ensure that he did not have malabsorption or blood loss. Russell's mother was seen by a paediatric dietitian to advise how to broaden his diet and include sources of iron to ensure he did not relapse.

Dental decay

Prevalence

In 1983, dental decay (caries) was seen in almost 50% of five-year-olds in the UK. Although there has been a dramatic reduction in the incidence of such since then, even now the average British 12-year-old has five decayed, filled or absent teeth.

Causes

Development of caries, though in part due to a genetic predisposition, is quite evidently strongly influenced by other factors such as sugar in the diet (especially sucrose – common table or cane sugar), poor oral hygiene (Fig. 8.7) and fluoride deficiency.

The process of caries starts when the protective outer shell of teeth – the enamel – is attacked and dissolved (demineralised). The destruction then spreads to the softer, sensitive part of the tooth beneath the enamel – the dentine – and the weakened enamel collapses to form a cavity. The tooth, unlike most (but not all) other tissues of the body, cannot repair itself.

Dietary sugars are the major cause of caries. Bacteria naturally occurring in the mouth metabolise sugars and produce lactic acid as a by-product of such. For caries to arise, sugar needs to be in direct contact with the tooth over a sufficient period

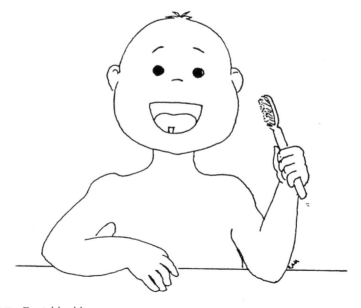

Figure 8.7   Dental health.

to allow the bacteria-produced acid to attack the enamel. It is for this reason that sugar in drinks is less cariogenic (causing caries) than the carbohydrates in sticky confectionery, cakes and toffee, which are adherent and potentially more harmful.

Prevention

Infants ought to be weaned onto foods, snacks and drinks free from the so-called non-milk extrinsic (NME) sugars (i.e. those other than lactose). Moreover, all children's medications ought to be sugar-free (*BMJ* editorial, 1995). Also, cup feeding should replace bottle-feeding after the age of one year, and drinks of soy formula between meals or at bedtime are not recommended. Soy drinks, which are not infant formulas, should not be used during weaning. They are deficient in energy and vitamins as well as calcium – unless they are fortified.

Carers should remove sweets, biscuits, etc. from the diet and substitute with milk or cheese for snacks. The caries-protective effect of cheese is well established. However, many parents do not wish to impose a harsh restrictive regimen on their children. A compromise would be to allow the forbidden foods on one day a week only, and for the teeth to be brushed before the eating of sticky sweets, to lower the concentration of mouth bacteria, and then following the eating of the chocolate bar(s) or similar 'treat', to remove some of the residual sticky sugars.

The role of fluoride in the prevention of dental caries is well proven. When domestic water supplies contain a concentration of one part per million (1 ppm) (100 g fluoride per 100 ml water), this disorder is reduced by over 50%. The Royal College of Physicians has recommended that domestic water be fluoridated with 1 ppm. A telephone call to the local water supply board is the quickest way to determine the fluoride content in the area. The British Dental Association advises a fluoride intake of 0.25 mg a day from two weeks to two years of age. The British Association for the Study of Community Dentistry recommends supplements from six months – in infants below this age, the concentrations of fluoride in human milk and formula are sufficient to meet their needs. Ingested fluoride drops/ tablets are more effective than fluoride in toothpaste.

Where the local water supply has less than 0.3 ppm of fluoride, reduction in caries will be achieved with daily fluoride supplements as recommended below:

- Age two weeks to two years, give 0.25 mg a day.
- Age two to four years, give 0.50 mg a day.
- Age four to 16 years, give 1.0 mg a day.

Theoretically, it is possible for small children who brush their teeth twice a day with fluorinated toothpaste and also receive this mineral in their water supply, to receive too much fluoride. Excess fluoride (e.g. >10 ppm in domestic water) can cause mottling of the dental enamel. Toothpaste should not contain more than 1000 ppm. Because the amount of fluoride that causes mottling is not much greater than the daily recommended amount, parents should be cautious, and add just small amounts (size of a small pea) of supplemented toothpaste to the brush, and only give drops or tablets when fully aware of the local water content.

In India, excess fluoride (fluorosis) is a major health problem – 25 million people suffer from too much of this element in their drinking water.

An encouraging future development, of interest to researchers in the field of paediatric dentistry, could be the development of a vaccine to prevent the presence in the mouth of *Streptococcus mutans*, the bacterium responsible for plaque formation.

Further reading
Cot death

- Gunther M (1977) Rearing human infants: breast or bottle? In: M Peakes (ed) *Comparative Aspects of Lactation*. Academic Press, London.

Food allery (food intolerance)

- Committee on Toxicology of Chemicals in Food, Consumer Products and the Environment (2000) *Adverse Reactions to Food and Food Ingredients*. Food Standards Agency, London.
- Leung DYM, Sampson HA, Geha RS *et al* (2003) *Pediatric Allergy*. Mosby, St Louis.
- Shaw V and Lawson M (2001) *Clinical Paediatric Dietetics*. Blackwell Scientific Publications, Oxford.
- Wright T (2001) *Food Allergies*. Class Publishing, London.

Additives and hyperkinesis

- Consumers' Association (1988) *Understanding Additives*. Which? Books, Consumers' Association and Hodder & Stoughton, London.
- Hanssen M (1984) *E for Additives*. Thorsons, Wellingborough.

Obesity

- Barlow SE and Dietz WH (1998) Obesity evaluation and treatment: expert committee recommendations. *Pediatrics* **102**: E29.
- NHS Centre for Reviews and Dissemination (2002) The prevention and treatment of childhood obesity. *Effective Health Care* **7**(6).
- Scottish Intercollegiate Guidelines Network (April 2003) *Management of Obesity in Children and Young People*. SIGN publication number 69.

Heart disease

- Barker D (2003) *The Best Start in Life*. Century, London.

Faltering growth

- Underdown A (2000) When feeding fails. *Community Pract.* **73**: 713–14.
- Wright CM (2000) Children who fail to thrive. *Curr Paediatr.* **10**: 191–5.

Dental decay

- Anon (1995) Children's dental health and medicines that contain sugar. *BMJ* **311**: 141–2.
- Department of Health (2002) *Scientific Review of the Welfare Food Scheme.* Report on Health and Social Subjects No. 51. The Stationery Office, London.

CHAPTER 9

Topical nutritional issues

Food irradiation

Many issues in dietetics and nutrition can arouse strong emotive responses from parents – for example, that of additives and behaviour, or caries and fluoride – but few can equal the subject of food irradiation. From the time of the Second World War, with memories of Hiroshima and Nagasaki in Japan, and, more recently, Chernobyl, anxieties are expressed when the matter of ionising radiation and food is aired.

Food irradiation is the process of exposing food to a carefully controlled amount of ionising energy. The food is passed through a field of ionising energy from either machine-generated electron beams or gamma rays from cobalt-60. The ionising radiation passes through the food, generating large numbers of short-lived free radicals. These can kill micro-organisms, such as salmonella, and inhibit many processes, such as those that cause sprouting and ripening (Fig. 9.1). Irradiation of food by ultraviolet light will destroy some microbes on the surface of foods, but there is no penetration as is seen with ionising radiation.

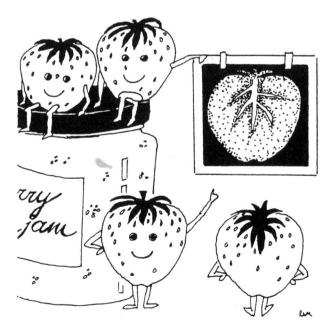

Figure 9.1 Irradiated food.

In the UK, the Advisory Committee on Irradiated and Novel Foods (ACINEF) approved irradiation in 1986 as a safe and satisfactory method of food processing. This opinion was reaffirmed in 1987 after receiving submissions from industry, consumer groups and interested parties. In 1991, the Food (Control of Irradiation) Regulations in the UK cleared seven categories of food for irradiation to the specified overall average doses:

- fruits (2.0 kGy)
- vegetables (1.0 kGy)
- cereals (1.0 kGy)
- bulbs and tubers (0.2 kGy)
- spices and condiments (10 kGy)
- fish and shellfish (3.0 kGy)
- poultry (7.0 kGy).

Under the Food Labelling Regulations (1996), irradiated foods and ingredients have to be identified with the words 'irradiated' or 'treated with ionising radiation'. Irradiation facilities must also meet specified criteria before they can be licensed to process foods. To date, the only licences granted within the UK have been for the treatment of certain spices.

The recommendation of a maximum overall average dose of 10 kGy (1 million rads) is currently under review. This level is in accordance with the conclusion of a Study Group convened in 1997 by the Joint Food and Agriculture Organization of the United Nations (FAO)/International Atomic Energy Agency (IAEA)/World Health Organisation (WHO), which commented that this dosage does not present any toxological risk. Moreover, the Expert Committee expressed the view that the irradiation of food did not introduce either nutritional or microbiological hazard. A similar judgment has been made by the Board of the International Committee on Food Microbiology and Hygiene of the International Union of Microbiological Societies. Although there is a considerable body of opinion assuring the public that there is no danger in the procedure of food irradiation, it has been claimed that the various expert organisations and those with vested interests have failed to note public concern in the UK about this issue (Webb and Lang, London Food Commission).

Chromosome defects have been reported in malnourished children fed on irradiated wheat, but the evidence has been said to be equivocal and inadequate to justify withholding a food irradiation programme. An ACINEF report concluded that the defects were transient.

One important plus point for the use of food irradiation is the removal of Salmonella from chickens after their slaughter. This microbe is a common and major source of food-poisoning outbreaks. Such a policy would be a great boost to improved public health standards, but some might view this suggested measure as too simplistic and be concerned over the potential use of the technology to cover up unhygienic food production.

Genetically modified (GM) foods

Food has been modified for centuries. In the past this was done by selective breeding. For example, farmers would take the seeds of cereals that were not damaged by, perhaps, a fungus, and propagate them to produce a strain relatively more resistant to fungi. Others would develop giant pumpkins and strains of wheat with a high degree of resistance to known diseases. Farm animals might be selectively bred for specific and desirable qualities.

Genetic engineering techniques enable scientists to insert specific genes into plants or animals without incurring the long delays in time and expense that they would previously have encountered; for example, a gene that produces a natural insecticide could be implanted into corn to eliminate damage from corn borers. Also, genetic engineering allows the scientist to cross species very easily and so a plant can be developed to produce human insulin.

Most infant formulas do not contain GM ingredients.

Probiotics and prebiotics

The normal microflora in the gastrointestinal tract has been described as 'a rich ecosystem'. Microbial colonisation takes place during birth. The newborn is inoculated with micro-organisms from the intestine and vaginal flora of the mother. Subsequently, there is a diverse bowel flora, which includes bifidobacteria, enterobacteria, *Bacteroides* species, clostridia and gram-positive cocci.

In breastfed babies – unlike in those fed on formula – bifidobacteria constitute more than 90% of the flora. This is in part due to the presence in human milk of 1% neutral oligosaccharides and 0.1% acidic oligosaccharides. Bifidobacteria provide a more beneficial intestinal environment by offering a lower pH and improving host resistance to pathogens by activation of the immune system.

Probiotics are food supplements consisting of live micro-organisms, thought to benefit health by improving the balance of microbes in the intestines. Most human consumption of probiotics is in the form of yoghurts and other dairy products containing lactobacilli and bifidobacteria.

Antibiotics, particularly if given long term, will upset the natural balance of the intestinal microflora. Probiotic foods and dietary supplements have been recommended as treatments for a variety of diseases and disorders, ranging from problems confined to the digestive tract to general health issues.

Probiotics and prebiotics modulate the composition of the intestinal microflora to the benefit of the host. A prebiotic is a compound (usually a carbohydrate such as an oligosaccharide) that reaches the colon and selectively favours the growth of lactic acid bacteria.

Aluminium contamination of infant formulas

The topic of aluminium in infant formulas attracted so much media attention in the UK at one point that soy-based formulas suddenly, albeit temporarily, disappeared from retail sources. A group of academic nutritionists wrote a letter to *The Lancet* (4 March 1989) reporting the high levels of aluminium to be found in cow's milk as compared with human milk, and the even greater quantities present in soy-based formulas. Breast milk has 5–20 μg/1 of aluminium, but in soy-based milks it is as much as 100-fold greater. A European Union Directive specifies that drinking water ought not to exceed a level of 200 μg/l. No sooner had the letter appeared in this distinguished international journal than anxious parents felt compelled to discard their soy milks — only to learn that other specific cow's milks have a range of aluminium stretching from 88 μg/l (e.g. SMA White) to 225 μg/l (Osterfeed Complete Formula).

The key to the mystery is that aluminium is the most abundant metal in the earth's crust, and tap water, which is used by the formula producers, contains a variable level of such, in England ranging from 100 μg/l to 300 μg/l; in north-west England, it can at times be much higher. The pitch of fear among parents — and, perhaps, doctors too — has been exacerbated by the awareness that aluminium toxicity may be linked with the development of Alzheimer's disease, a severe progressive dementia, although this association has not, as yet, been shown conclusively. There are insufficient data to show that any harm has befallen the tens, perhaps hundreds, of thousands of babies fed high-aluminium-containing milk preparations, to justify abandoning current feeding practice. Clearly, those babies with impaired renal function, i.e. premature newborns and low birthweight (LBW) babies, ought to avoid soy milk. Indeed, this was the recommendation made some years ago by the Committee of Nutrition of the American Academy of Pediatrics to those wanting to avoid the risk of later allergy in LBW and premature babies.

Finally, perhaps we can be reassured by noting a piece of recent research. This showed that healthy term infants under three months of age fed soy-based formulas, containing amounts of aluminium several-fold greater than those in human milk, had blood levels of this metal similar to those in breastfed infants. However, other risks are linked to soy-based formula (*see* Chapter 2).

Food poisoning

Food poisoning comprises a group of illnesses varying in severity from mild and self-limited to life-threatening, due to ingestion of contaminated food (Fig. 9.2). Various micro-organisms may cause it, the most common being pathogenic bacteria or their products (toxins) (*see* Table 9.1).

Listeriosis and food

Listeria is a microbe that is well known to both veterinary surgeons and paediatricians because of the diseases it can cause in animals and children following consumption of contaminated foods. *L. monoctogenes*, a significant pathogen for humans, has been found in 37 different types of animals and more than 17 species of birds. The two groups of the population most at risk are pregnant women and those with a compromised immune system (e.g. those with AIDS, leukaemia and patients on steroids, etc.). Although this microbe can cause very serious disease, it is pertinent to remember that one in 20 of the population have Listeria in their bowel with no ill effects. This organism has the uncommon property of being able to multiply at temperatures which may be found in the domestic refrigerator (6°C or above). Foods, particularly if they are consumed without needing to be cooked, are an important source of infection.

Listeria has been found with high bacterial counts in pasteurised as well as unpasteurised milk, and can be traced to both cows and goats. Soft ripened cheeses

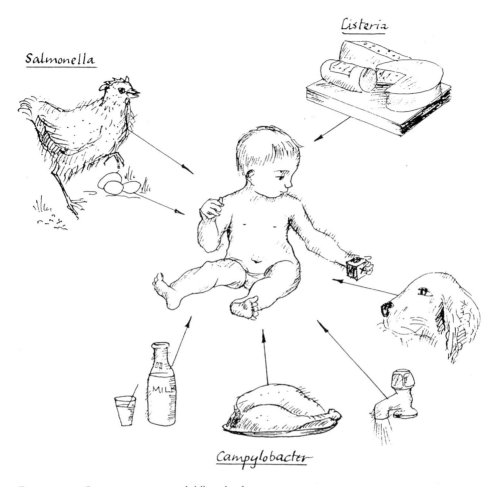

Figure 9.2   Current anxieties in childhood infection.

(e.g. Brie, Camembert, blue-vein types) are one source of Listeria. Hardened cheeses (e.g. Cheddar and Cheshire type), processed cheeses, cottage cheeses and cheese spreads have not given cause for concern. Other sources include pre-cooked ready-to-eat poultry, and cooked and chilled meats – these require reheating to a very high temperature (throughout the food) before being eaten.

Pregnant women and others who are vulnerable must reheat all foods thoroughly and use careful standards of hygiene when handling pre-packed salads, which can be contaminated with Listeria. They should avoid all unpasteurised milk and dairy products. A pregnant woman might have a vague flu-like illness or a subclinical infection, and not be aware of her true problem; as a consequence, the listeriosis may not be diagnosed or treated promptly or properly to protect her foetus or newborn. Infection of the foetus might be responsible for spontaneous abortion, stillbirth or the birth of a desperately ill baby. In 1988 in England and Wales there were 11 miscarriages, nine stillbirths and six neonatal deaths (during the first 28 days of life) from this cause, although listeriosis is still a rare disease.

Table 9.1   Agents responsible for food poisoning.

Agent	Food sources
Salmonella sp.	Raw meat, poultry, raw milk (cow, goat or sheep), eggs; also, rarely, from a tropical fish tank
Clostridium perfringens	Meat, poultry, dried foods, herbs, spices, vegetables
Staphylococcus aureus	Cold foods, dairy products (especially if prepared from raw milk)
Escherichia coli	Many raw foods and milk
Vibrio parahaemolyticus	Raw and cooked fish, shellfish and other seafoods (Japanese restaurants are one potential source)
Yersinia enterocolitica	Raw meat and poultry, milk, milk products, vegetables (well-described from Belgian sources)
Campylobacter jejuni	Raw poultry, meat, raw or inadequately heat-treated milk, untreated water
Listeria monocytogenes	Meat, poultry, dairy products (especially soft blue-vein cheeses), vegetables and shellfish
Viruses	Raw shellfish, cold foods prepared by infected food handlers

Eggs and salmonellosis

Salmonellas are one of the major causes of food-borne illnesses throughout the world. In the UK and many other Western countries, reported cases of salmonellosis have increased markedly in the last decade. The principal symptoms of infection include diarrhoea, abdominal pain, fever, etc. Contaminated food and water are often responsible for the infection. Usually there are few if any problems in the host carrier, but the microbes are found in large numbers in the stools.

Although there are more than 1000 types of salmonellas, virtually all of which can cause human disease, recent UK attention has focused upon one specific serotype – *Salmonella enteritidis* 4. Because poultry farm food may be contaminated with this particular microbe, it can then be transferred to hens' eggs and finally the consumer.

Awareness of the frequency in the UK of this specific form of food poisoning has led to the government issuing guidelines warning children (and others too) not to eat raw eggs and emphasising the importance of cooking eggs to a high temperature – so, if boiled, they are hard, and similarly, if scrambled or fried, they must be well-cooked – in order to destroy the organism if present.

Revelations about the hazard of egg eating hit a peak in the UK in 1988. The political dialogue became so intense that a junior government minister was obliged to resign because she was accused of overstating the prevalence of the problem. Subsequently, egg sales plummeted so severely in the UK that the government was lobbied to introduce financial compensation for the egg farmers. An inevitable consequence was that the public would soon realise that if eggs were the secondary source of food poisoning, then chickens were also a risk to the consumer as they were the primary origin. Contamination of poultry is not limited to salmonellas, however; another potentially dangerous organism, *Campylobacter jejuni*, is found in milk and poultry as well as in domestic animals.

The avoidance and control of salmonellosis requires preventive action by the catering trade, agriculture and food industry as well as by the consumer of and, more importantly, the preparer of foods. This is especially meaningful when considering restaurants, communal/hospital kitchens and the catering industry. Hygienic abattoir practices are of the utmost priority with regard to the content of salmonellas in meat.

Unless meat abattoirs are carefully inspected – and some would much rather that this was done by veterinary surgeons who are highly qualified and not by environmental health officers (viz. the UK, c.f. elsewhere in Western Europe) – then there is a risk that the perforated bowel of a cow's carcass might contaminate the animal's tissues with faecal material and pose a health hazard. Without adequate numbers of health inspectors, better food hygiene, education and the financial resources all that entails, then poultry and eggs, meat and milk, and indeed fish too, will continue to play a major role in the cause of childhood food poisoning. The Food Standards Agency has developed a 'farm-to-fork' strategy to meet its target of reducing food poisoning by 20% by 2006.

Bovine spongiform encephalopathy (BSE)

BSE – a fatal prion disease of adult cattle – was first noted in the UK in 1985. Since then, more than 170 000 confirmed cases have been identified in British cattle.

The disorder originates from the spinal cord and brain of infected cattle and can pass between animals of the same species. The key question is whether it can be transmitted to humans. One important control measure taken in the late 1980s was the removal of certain offal from bovine carcasses to reduce the risk of eventual transmission to beef eaters.

The subject has become more diffuse because a similar, potentially fatal degenerative neurological disorder, Creutzfeldt-Jakob disease (CJD), has been described in several UK farmers. Thus, one of the many questions posed by this controversy is whether CJD is linked to BSE in infected cattle, or, perhaps, scrapie. The latter is a brain disease of sheep and goats endemic in many countries and recorded in the UK for well over 200 years. Despite the reassuring comments of government spokespersons, it is disquieting to note that all four UK farmers who died from CJD in 1995 each had at least one infected cow in his herd. As yet, the jury is still out in respect of suspected links between BSE and CJD. However, as a result of media attention and perhaps irrational yet understandable fears, there has been an inevitable fall in meat consumption.

Risks to immigrant communities

Surma and lead poisoning

Where family practitioners are caring for immigrant communities, a specific awareness of potential hazards when families return home on vacation is important. An example is the use of Surma (Soorma), a black powder often imported from East Africa or India that might contain lead or antimony. It is used for staining the baby's eyelashes or eyebrows in some communities. Application to the skin might result in plumbism.

Arsenic and well water supplies

Families returning to Bangladesh need reminding that drinking water from sunken wells might have a very high content of this poison. Half the population of Bangladesh and many in West Bengal are at risk of arsenic poisoning.

Further reading

- Kumar S (2003) Millions more at risk of arsenic poisoning than previously thought. *BMJ.* **326**: 466.

Recommendations for energy intake

Age	Estimated average intake[1]	
	kcal/kg/day	kJ/kg/day
1 month	115	480
3 months	100	420
6–36 months	95	400
Males:		
3 years	97	405
4 years	94	395
5 years	88	370
6 years	84	350
7 years	78	325
Females:		
3 years	92	385
4 years	87	365
5 years	82	345
6 years	71	320
7 years	66	295
	kcal/day	MJ/day
Males:		
7–10 years	1970	8.24
11–14 years	2200	9.27
15–18 years	2755	11.51
Females:		
7–10 years	1740	7.28
11–14 years	1845	7.92
15–18 years	2110	8.33

[1] From Dietary Reference Values for Food Energy and Nutrients for the United Kingdom. Department of Health Report on Health and Social Subjects No. 41. London: HMSO, 1991. Estimated Average Requirement.

APPENDIX 2

Recommendations for protein intake

Age	$g/kg/day$[1]
0–3 months	2.10
4–6 months	1.65
7–9 months	1.55
10–12 months	1.54
1–3 years	1.16
4–6 yers	1.11
7–10 years	1.00

	g/day
Males:	
11–14 years	42.10
15–18 years	55.20
Females:	
11–14 years	43.80
15–18 years	45.40

[1]From Dietary Reference Values for Food Energy and Nutrients for the United Kingdom. Department of Health Report on Health and Social Subjects No. 41. London: HMSO, 1991. Estimated Average Requirement.

APPENDIX 3

Normal fluid requirements

Age	Weight (kg)	Fluid per day
Preterm	1–2	150–200 ml/kg
0–6 months	2–8	120–150 ml/kg
7–12 months	6–10	100–120 ml/kg
	11–20	1000 ml + 50 ml/kg for each additional kg over 10 kg
	>20	1500 ml + 25 ml/kg for each additional kg over 20 kg (to a max. of 2500 ml/day)

Girls' preterm growth chart – 30 weeks' gestation to 52 weeks

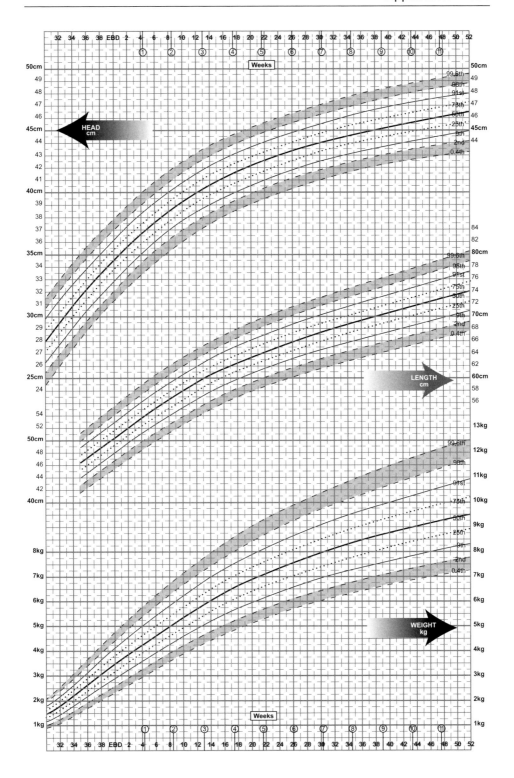

Boys' preterm growth chart – 30 weeks' gestation to 52 weeks

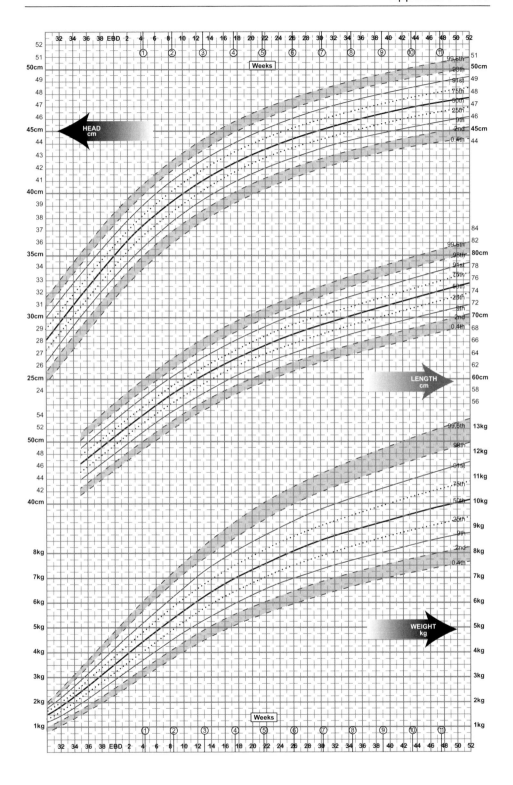

Girls' growth chart
12–24 months

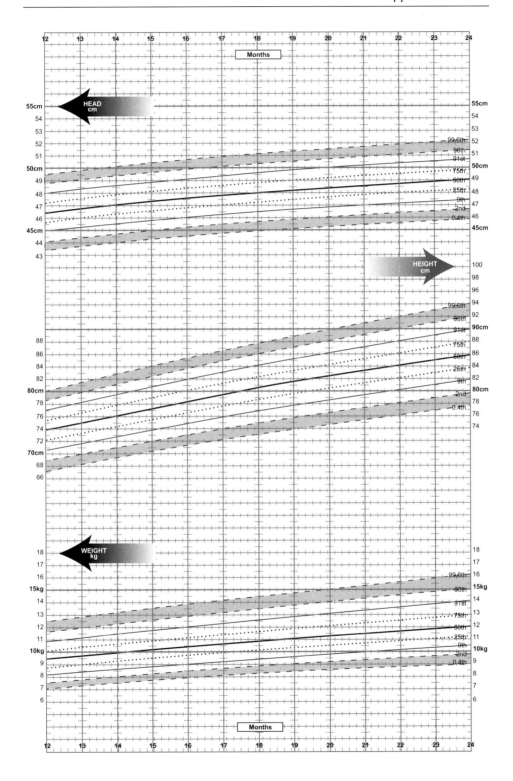

Boys' growth chart
12–24 months

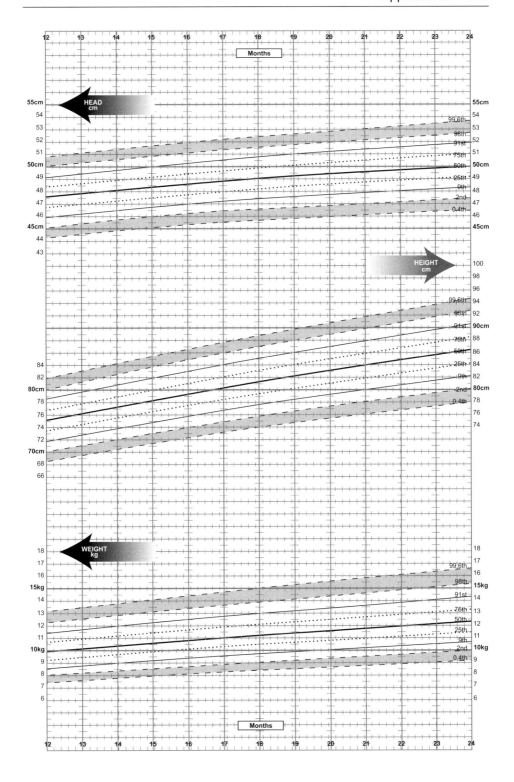

Girls' BMI chart
(birth to 20 years)

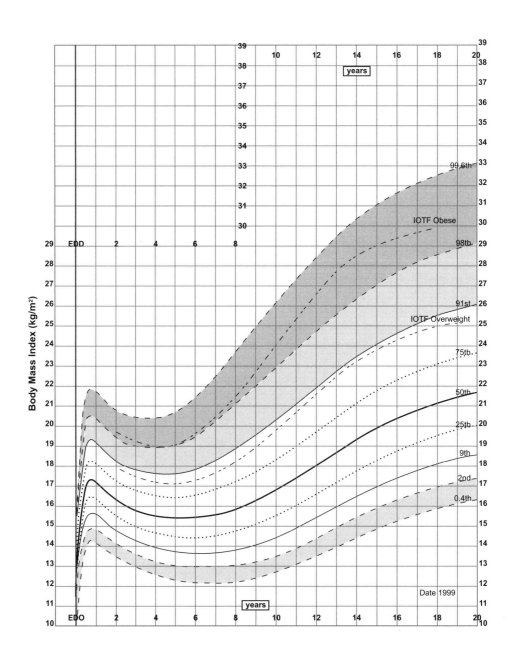

Boys' BMI chart (birth to 20 years)

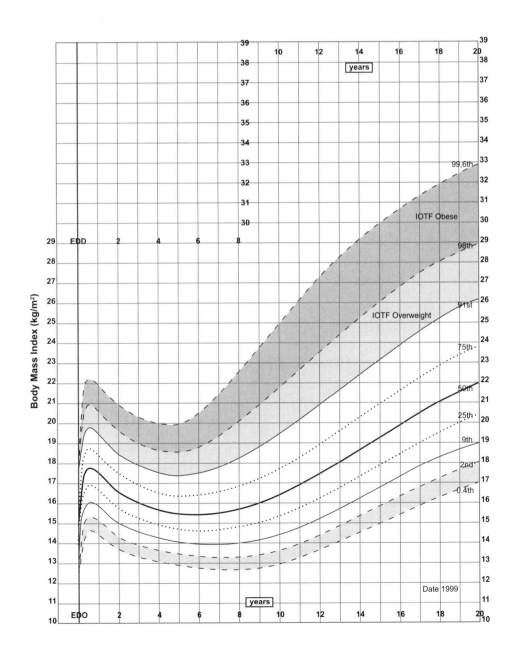

Index

Radcliffe Publishing Ltd

18 Marcham Road
Abingdon, Oxon
OX14 1AA, UK

+44 (0)1235 528820
+44 (0)1235 528830
contact.us@radcliffemed.com
www.radcliffe-oxford.com

Infant Feeding and Nutrition in Primary Care – Erratum

On page 35, Nan HA has incorrectly been classified as a Therapeutic Infant Formula.

Nan H.A. is indicated for use in non-breast fed healthy infants who have a predisposition to developing cow milk protein intolerance. This whey based and only partially hydrolysed product is contraindicated in those with an intolerance to cow's milk proteins.

with compliments